THE FABULOUS BODY

BUILD LEAN MUSCLE, SHED BODY FAT & OPTIMIZE YOUR HEALTH

AKASH SEHRAWAT, HHP, CPT

FABULOUS BODY INC

Cover designed by Subrato Deb
Edited by Maria Kuzmiak (www.wellbeingwriter.net)

For my son Vince

CONTENTS

TOP 9 REASONS WHY YOU SHOULD READ THIS BOOK

1. You want to build lean and proportionate muscles but don't want to look like a bodybuilder. I have gone from 140 pounds to 178 pounds (current) and I don't look like one; neither will you. The idea is to have enough muscles to keep people interested but not so much to scare them off.

2. You want to drop your body fat and bring it into the optimal range (for men, 9 to 14 percent; for women, 19 to 24 percent). I don't support an extreme ripped look with body fat in the low single digits.

3. You want to build a pleasant looking body that is also functional and optimally healthy. The Fabulous Body training system (FBX) is a multifaceted system that ensures you develop a well-rounded physique.

4. You are serious about your health and fitness goals but have limited time. FBX optimizes your gene expression in only 3 – 6 hours per week. You don't need to do more.

5. You have limited funds to allocate to your health and fitness goals. FBX can be pursued with very basic equipment, including home gyms. Further, the Reality Diet (a term I used for a no-fad diet—notice it's not FAT but FAD) focuses on home-made meals with very little use of supplements.

6. You want to cut through the pseudo and bro science, which is rather overwhelming and confusing for most of us. This book provides you the "truth" that the

conventional sources (supplement companies, muscle and fitness magazines) are hiding from you.

7. You are not looking for mere opinions but rather hard scientific facts. This book is linked with more than 100 scientific studies to support any concept or theory discussed. All these concepts have been part of my lifestyle long enough for me to know whether they work or not. I will never discuss something just because it is popular or trending. Furthermore you don't need to imbibe (or even believe) everything I say. I would be delighted if you internalize even a single idea from this book that pays you handsomely in long run.

8. You don't just need a book but a system, a workbook where you simply plug in and start your workouts immediately. Fabulous Body is a paradigm with three pillars and nine laws that will act as a personal coach in your quest to build your dream physique. Further, there are 16 FBX printable workout routines in the added FREE BONUS REPORT that will get you started right off the bat. These workouts are divided into beginner, intermediate and advanced levels. They are further sub-divided into FBX-Cut and FBX-Gain to help you build muscles and lose fat efficiently and effectively.

9. You are open-minded. You have the courage to try something new or even radical and not simply follow what other people are doing in the gym.

PREFACE

Hi, I am Akash, and I am the creator of fabulousbody.com.

My mission is to **Empower**, **Educate** and **Inspire** you to build a fabulous body that not only looks **Pleasing** but is also **Functional** and **Healthy**.

I suffered by following conventional wisdom and almost gave up my dream of building my ideal physique. I work very hard to filter out the DUST (pseudo and bro science) and provide you with clear, specific, and credible information that will help you build lean muscles, drop body fat and optimize your health in the most cost effective, timely, and natural way possible.

I am a Holistic Health Practitioner with a Doctor of Naturopathy from Indian Board of Alternative Medicines. I also have two certifications from the National Academy of Sports Medicine (NASM)—certified personal trainer and performance enhancement specialist. I have more than a decade of experience in the fitness industry and have been running my own health club since 2010.

Now, you should know that I AM NOT A PROFESSIONAL WRITER, nor did I hire a ghostwriter to write this book. I asked to my dear editor Maria to edit the book in a way that made sure I didn't lose my tone and voice, and this whole book should seem like a long personalized email from a friend. In the end, I feel Maria has done a great job.

How this book is structured

For your ease, I have categorized the book into three sections: The Basics, Training, and Nutrition. In the basics section, I start off by explaining the personal circumstances that led me to create Fabulous Body. After that, I explain what Fabulous Body is, describe its laws, and then give you the five specific steps to for building one. Next, you will learn about the four mindset principles that will almost guarantee your success. In the next chapters, I talk about the REAL science behind muscle building and fat loss.

Next, comes the Training part. Here I will introduce you to the Fabulous Body Training System: **FBX**. I discuss in depth the various training variables that bring a workout together. Once you understand these, you will have the tools to easily customize your own workouts according to your individualized needs and goals. I have also listed 16 FBX printable workout routines that will get you started ASAP. They can be found in the FREE bonus report you will get with this book.

The last chapter of the Training section is an important one on how to get the most out of your workout. I feel most people have an abundance of motivation to build a good body but lack conviction or courage to maneuver through the commercial gym environment. Reading this chapter will help you maximize your workout output dramatically.

Next, in the nutrition section, you will read about what I call "The Reality Diet," a type of diet that is not restrictive and is based on key nutritional guidelines and principles. My in-depth discussion on the macronutrients will help you choose them in the right ratio according to your body type. I further discuss the concept of intermittent fasting and provide you with my weekly diet plan and my ingredient list. Last but not the least, I discuss the topmost effective supplements I use to maximize my results.

INTRODUCTION

We live in a world of ideas. In his book, *Unleashing the Ideavirus*, Seth Godin states, "We recognize that ideas are driving the economy, ideas are making people rich and most important, ideas are changing the world."

My physique has been completely transformed by a collection of key ideas I have implemented over the past few years. I have gained more than 20 pounds of lean, proportionate muscles and dropped my body fat from around 22-25 percent to somewhere between 12-15 percent. In addition to my tremendous gains in lean muscle and tone, I have moved towards experiencing optimal health. Here are some of the radical changes I made to my lifestyle:

1. I reduced my workout frequency from five to six times per week to just two to three times per week, saving myself around ten hours per week.

2. I've gone from eating five or six small meals a day to just two or three meals a day. This again helps me to save more time while optimizing my health. I love the concept of intermittent fasting, which I discuss in the nutrition section.

3. I have made a massive increase in the percent of calories I consume from fat sources, jumping from 15 percent to 30 percent. Sometimes, I even go as high as 40 percent. People don't realize that healthy fats are actually good for you and that one should eat fat to burn fat. I'll give you all the details about this in the nutrition section.

4. I have not let a single week pass without allowing myself a cheat meal, including heavy buffets and the occasional mug of beer, glass of wine, or dessert. Who said you have leave out your favorite foods in order to build your dream physique?

5. I have substantially decreased my use of nutritional supplements—most of them are worthless—opting for just the most effective ones and saving myself at least a few hundred dollars per month. My supplementation guide in Chapter 22 will assist you in doing the same.

"Everything that is popular is wrong!" Oscar Wilde

My approach is more radical than that of most experts out there.

This book is essentially a collection of RADICAL IDEAS that will set you free from all the information overload and misguided conventional wisdom.

The information in this book has been carefully selected. I have spent many years assembling it. I don't think anyone reading this wants to spend more than ten years on trial and error or thousands of dollars on certifications, scientific books, and journals and then relentlessly apply the principles to see what works and what doesn't. Unless you plan to make a career out of it, reading my book is a much easier way to get what you want.

I promise you will be completely transformed in about six months to a year if you follow my program with dedication. You will be amazed by how much your body can change in so little time simply by making smart choices every day.

Now, if you're looking for some kind of shortcut, I am not your man. But, if you are willing to put some time and effort into following my FBX training system, you will:

- ☐ Be able to build up to 10-15 pounds of dense, rock hard muscle (even more if you are a beginner/intermediate) within six months to a year.

- ☐ Be able to easily drop your body fat and bring it into the ideal range.

- ☐ Achieve a 'classic' body that people will stop in their tracks to admire or even earn appreciative glances when you take off your clothes at the beach or pool.

- ☐ Experience fewer (or no) headaches, migraines, and digestive problems (and you'll probably start to wonder why these chronic ailments affect so many people!) and be well on your way towards optimizing your health.

- ☐ Amaze your family and friends with your transformation in the fastest time possible.

- ☐ Find unlimited energy and easily work ten hours a days with relentless focus if you desire.

The concepts, tools, and strategies in this book are not new. In fact, they are timeless principles that have been applied to shape thousands of fabulous physiques over the years. I am simply someone who stumbled upon them, diligently researched them, relentlessly applied them for a few years, and saw tremendous results.

I'm not an innovator; I'm simply a messenger.

SECTION 1: THE BASICS

CHAPTER 1:
THE VAST MAJORITY OF YOUR SOURCES ARE WRONG

Before we go further, I want you try this five-minute exercise:

Go to a place where no one will disturb you. Close your eyes, take a few deep breaths, and ask yourself these questions:

1. Do you like the way you look right now, either naked or with your favorite jeans and shirt on? Does your slim-fit Zara shirt fit perfectly, or you are conscious of your protruding belly all the time?

2. Are you having a really hard time getting rid of the body fat from your belly or face?

3. Every time you go to a party or a get-together, do you promise yourself that you will look your best at the next one? How long have you been saying that?

4. When you get up in the morning, committed to changing your lifestyle, does something get in your way, such as your family, job, or other commitments?

5. Do you like to stay in your comfort zone?

6. Did you once dream of building a physique similar to your favorite celebrity, but now you are simply settling for "staying in shape"?

Now, open your eyes and stand in front of a full-length mirror. WHAT DO YOU SEE?
Do you see someone who has failed you miserably in the past few months or years?

Do you see someone who makes tall promises all the time and never really takes action to accomplish them?

I'm sorry for making you feel like that. Now, let's look at the bright side, shall we?

When something is not right and we want to change our circumstances—whether it's related to our looks, our health, our financial status, or even our relationships—**the fact that we want to make improvements is a very positive sign.**

Use this energy, this feeling, and these circumstances to propel yourself forward.

Now, I want to make one thing clear: **I don't completely blame YOU for the condition you are in.**

With billion and billions of dollars being spent on useless products—miracle weight loss pills, fancy cutting-edge protein supplements, and ever more "perfect" programs promoted to lure you in—**I believe you have been fed a big lie.**

These guys—the supplement companies and popular health and fitness magazines—are laughing all the way to the bank, and you're helping them do so by blindly trusting them.

Conventional wisdom is confusing you. Its proponents want to keep things mysterious and interesting. Think of it as being like our 24/7 news channels. There isn't much solid content to show on the news for just a few hours a day, let alone 24/7, but the news channels need to show something. So what do they do? They dramatize the smallest things and show them repeatedly with a twist to keep things interesting.

In my experience in the fitness industry, I've observed that most people get their information regarding fitness, nutrition, and health from two main sources:

1. Popular fitness and muscle magazines (or websites)
2. Fitness trainers

Popular fitness and muscle magazines (or websites)

If there is a strong demand in the market for something, there will never be a scarcity of new, cutting edge products to fill that need. There will always be savvy marketers inventing the latest discoveries or some miracle diet, product, or training program. All of this new, interesting "research" and the so-called groundbreaking supplements are merely marketing tools designed to confuse you and fill up pages in the magazines with the main goal of selling more supplements.

If you pick up any fitness or bodybuilding magazine, you'll see what I mean right away.

Here are the three main problems with these magazines:

1. **They promote programs that are useless to the masses**. Most of the programs are geared toward champion bodybuilders who are on steroids and/or other drugs—people whose whole lives revolve around being in the gym. How can people like you and me, who have average genetics and tons of other responsibilities, possibly get results being on these programs, which require you to:
    - Be in the gym almost every day
    - Do a lot of isolated training and split routines
    - Rely on boatloads of supplements, including protein drinks, pre-workouts, glutamine, BCAAs, and God knows what else

2. **Their main mission is to sell supplements**. This fact is not surprising given that most of the supplement companies own the magazines. On almost every page, there is a full-page ad where a massive monster (no pun intended) is used to promote all sorts of supplements that are guaranteed to give you that ripped physique in no time.

3. **The information is confusing**. How many times have you realized that you are more confused after reading fitness magazines than you were before you read them? This is because the information is very isolated in its approach. Sure, you might learn a trick or two that helps you a little, but you never get a holistic view because the magazines want to be mysterious. After all, if you learn the truth and get results that way, how will the fitness magazines get you to buy more of their stuff?

Now, let's take a look at the other source that has conditioned your thinking:

Fitness trainers

I was a personal trainer myself before becoming an author, consultant, and entrepreneur.

I don't believe in pseudo science or "bro science" or the kinds of things you often find in newspapers and magazines.

Why is it that will you will find very few personal trainers like myself who keep abreast of the latest developments in exercise and nutrition science and continually upgrade their knowledge?

Here is the issue: No one wants to keep spending truckloads of money, time, and effort on continuing education.

Some of my friends are certified personal trainers, and they have very basic knowledge of anatomy and physiology. Can they be counted as experts? No! First of all, they don't keep up. Simply passing a certification exam doesn't make you a safe and effective trainer. You need to continually update your knowledge, which is a time-consuming and expensive ordeal.

Many trainers simply take their clients through some basic questionnaires that their gym provides; they calculate BMI and then suggest programs they have recently read about in a popular muscle/fitness magazine. These trainers may instruct clients to do an exercise that no one is doing in the gym (which is potentially harmful) and voila, their job is done!

Is this really fair to the poor client who shells out a hefty amount of their hard-earned money ($25-$75 per session)?

The truth is that most trainers only care about their own physique, and most of them are out of shape themselves!

Since 2010, I have been running a successful health club in Delhi-NCR, India, and I was a personal trainer in many gyms before that, so I can very well say with surety that the situation I've described is very, very common in gyms and in the fitness industry in general.

Having said that, there are still a few good trainers out there who have the best intentions and sincerely want to help you, but these trainers are very few in number, and you will be lucky if you come across one of them yourself!

CHAPTER 2:
HOW MY STRUGGLE WITH CONVENTIONAL WISDOM LED ME TO CREATE FABULOUS BODY

Everyone has different reasons for wanting to build their dream physique. For some it's about attracting the opposite sex, for some it's about improving self-esteem and building confidence, and for others it's all about vanity! I'll be the first to admit that vanity was my driving force initially, although my motivations have since evolved.

Quite simply, I was a teenage boy who wanted to fill his measly 33-inch chest with some brawn.

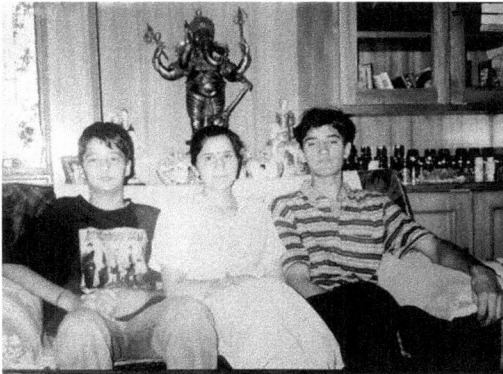

Vikki, Mom & Me

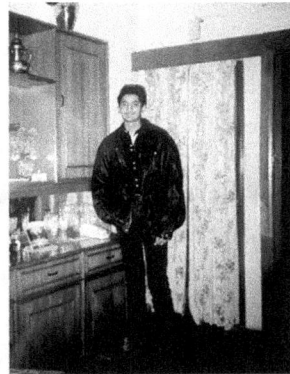

Notice how the weight of the jacket is pulling me down

I believe we are designed to go for things that we don't have, and we often become obsessive about that thing and view it as a "must" in our life. Without that drive, we would be unhappy and we might even perish.

What is that one thing in your life? Think about it.

Motivational coach Tony Robbins didn't have food to feed to his family. When someone knocked on his door and gave him food on Thanksgiving, it was a moment of reckoning for him. He is now the driving force behind the "**100 Million Meals Challenge**," which aims to provide free meals to children whose families cannot afford food. What an inspiration!

My Story

I decided to join a gym and pursue my passion of gaining muscle. My coaches at the time made me believe that it wouldn't be tough to do, and that I'd be a superman in no time. As an excited teenager with few responsibilities, I poured my heart and most of my free time into this passion.

There is a lot of conventional wisdom out there – you know, those generally accepted beliefs that you can find in nearly every book or website. It's what "they" say you should or shouldn't do, and these theories generally go unchallenged. This conventional wisdom told me a few things that I blindly followed, like

- ☐ Supplements build muscles - the more the better

- ☐ You should have more training days than rest days, and you should aim for higher volumes of isolated training. The more the better, "they" said.

- ☐ Muscle magazines are bibles, and one should blindly follow what champion bodybuilders do (without taking into account that some of them have better genetics working in their favor and most of them are on steroids).

What happened after ten years of applying this conventional bodybuilding wisdom? **DISAPPOINTMENT!**

I think these photos explain it all.

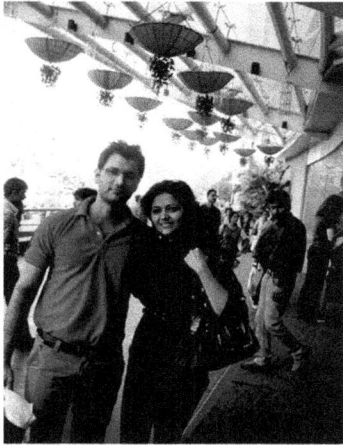

Me & Gia in 2010

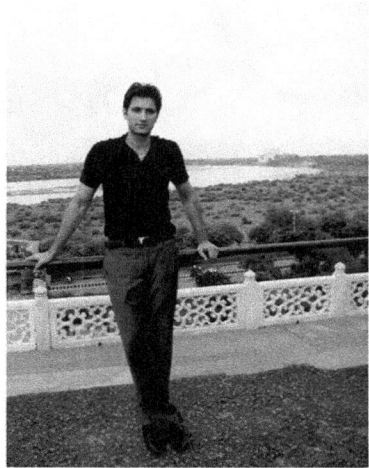

Me in 2012; still struggling to gain muscle

I thought I wasn't working hard enough to stimulate muscle building. I started training for two hours almost daily, eating around 3,500+ calories a day, and upping my supplement intake in a desperate attempt to gain some muscles.

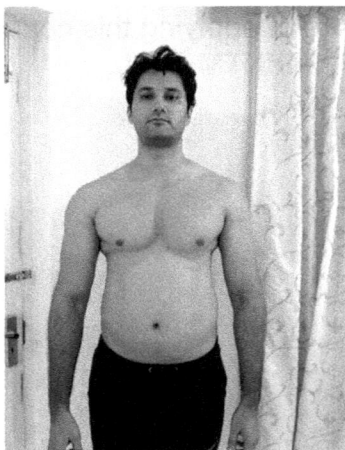

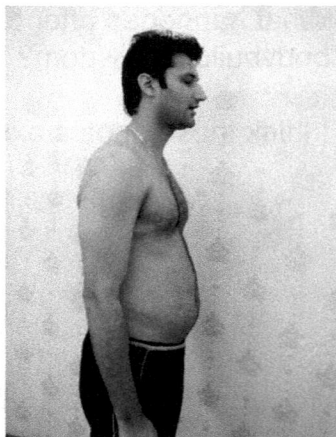

In a desperate attempt to gain muscle; instead gained 'tons of body fat' Year—2013

Eventually, I did indeed gain—but not much of it was muscles. It's close to impossible not to gain some muscles after so much training and following a good diet, but my idea of

building a dream physique is fulfilling my genetic potential. Building only 20 pounds of muscles in 10 long years along with tons of fat was not exactly what I had in mind.

Many people in the position I was in give up on the idea of building their dream physique, deeming it impossible. Instead, they resort to simply "staying in shape." Perhaps other things in life become priorities, and the need to impress everyone on the beach becomes an alien concept.

However, I realized one good thing about me. I did not simply give up on my quest to build my dream physique. I kept looking for answers!

Something I saw by accident changed my life.

You know, things that happen accidently can serve an important purpose in your life. They become a point at which in just one minute, your life changes as something inside of you transforms seemingly like the flick of a switch.

This is what happened in my case when **I saw a picture of Steve Reeves**. Boy, did he look good! I had never seen a more proportionate, symmetrical man in my life. Although he was big for his height, weighing 215 pounds (97 kg) at 6' 1" (185 cm), he never looked like those bodybuilding freaks that you see nowadays. I was blown away by his physique.

I was even more floored by something I read in Reeves' amazing book, *Building the Classic Physique*. He stated that he gained 30 pounds (13.6 kg) of solid muscle in just four months of training! He was only 16 years old at the time, and he did it without any supplements whatsoever (unless you count his homemade protein shakes). I immediately wished I had started following his program when I was 16. In fact, I would have been quite happy if I had gotten even half the results he did in the same timeframe!

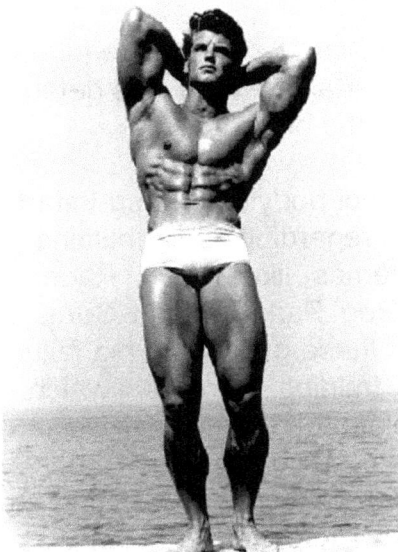

After digging deeper and applying Reeves' training principles, I finally saw some solid results. **For the first time in my life, I truly believed that my body had the capacity to gain muscles.** It felt good, but I still wasn't reaching my goal.

To be fair, Steve was just 16 when he achieved his classic physique, which meant he had high levels of HGH and testosterone and his recovery ability was at its peak. Moreover, he didn't have any other responsibilities distracting him from building his physique.

I realized that I needed a system that would give me mind-blowing results while considering my lifestyle and responsibilities at that time. After all, I had a wife and a child, I was over 30, and I worked more than 50 hours per week. I had a significantly higher amount of stress and responsibility than I'd had in my early 20s.

In order for a system to truly work for me, it would need to fit my lifestyle and schedule while also being financially feasible. I also wanted a program that required as few supplements as possible and employed only basic machinery and free weights. I wanted a program that I could eventually promote to the masses and not just the lucky few who have access to fancy gyms.

Perhaps the most important requirement was that my program be practical. To me, this meant no more than three to six hours of training in a week. **Let's face it—time is a major constraint for nearly everyone. We all lead busy lives.**

I knew that finding a program that fit all of my requirements would be a very ambitious undertaking, but I was determined to find something that would fit the bill.

Steve Reeves was an old-school bodybuilder, so I started to dig into older literature regarding weightlifting and bodybuilding. I turned to names like Peary Rader, Bob Hoffman, Stuart McRobert, Reg Park, Joseph Curtis Hise, and John McCallum. A few of these guys were big failures in the early stages of their training careers, which was something I could certainly relate to!

I read hundreds of books, newsletters, articles, and stories about these iron men. **What struck me the most was that they accomplished their results before the steroid era.** Steroids were introduced after the 1960s, which was when bodybuilding shifted from being a health-oriented sport to being a drug-oriented one. I started to figure out what could work for me given my preconditions (average genetics, being in my 30s, and having tons of responsibilities).

I took the patterns that started to emerge and combined them with the latest scientific knowledge and the practicalities of the modern lifestyle. I was desperate to get results this time. After ten years of failure, I was literally on the brink of giving up and probably would have convinced myself to accept that it was simply my fate to never gain enough muscles. I embarked on what was basically a last-ditch effort, but finally my **persistence** paid off!

Not only did I get results, but my progress went through the roof!

After following this program for the last few years, here is my current physique:

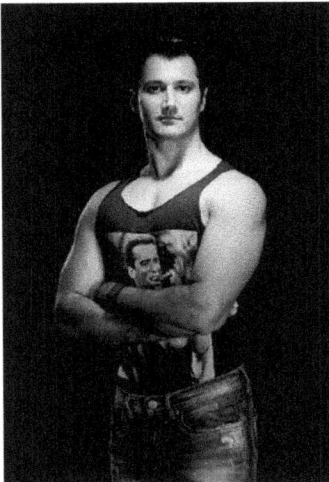

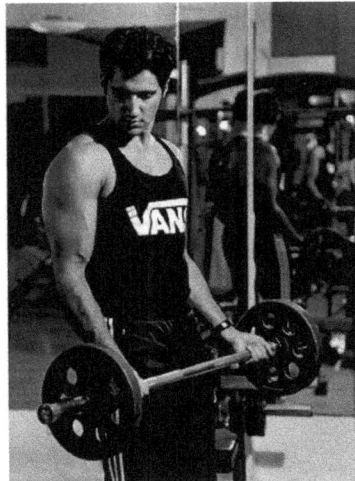

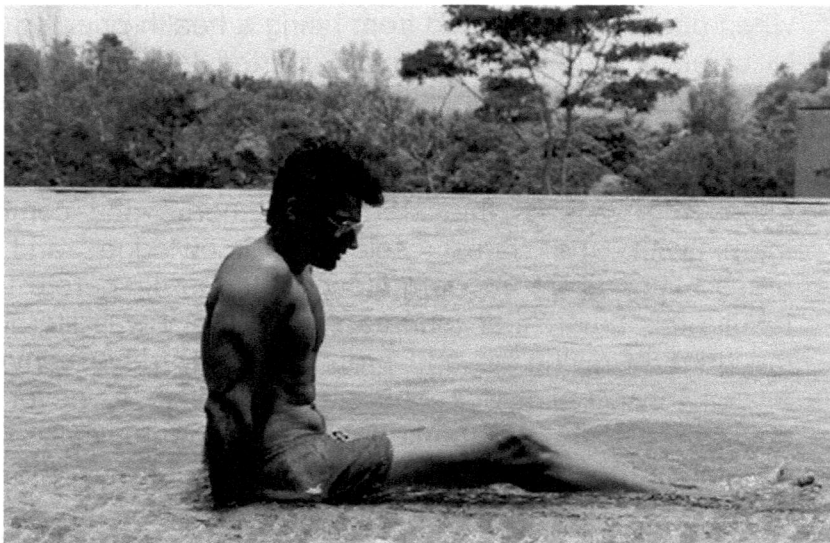

They say experience is the most convincing teacher, and I've managed to convince myself and others after gaining more than 40 pounds of rock-solid lean mass so far (my target is 60 pounds) with barely any fat gain. Most of my gains have come in the last few years, after I ditched conventional wisdom and instead discovered the **truth** about what works.

CHAPTER 3:
WHAT IS A FABULOUS BODY?

A "Fabulous Body" is a physique that is not only pleasing to look at but is also functional and optimally healthy. Achieving it is based on three pillars and nine fundamental laws.

Let's discuss these pillars and laws briefly.

THE THREE PILLARS OF A FABULOUS BODY

REAL: Fabulous bodies are real. They are not built out of an obsession with six-pack abs or an extreme ripped look. Every muscle is purposefully built to be in proportion to the rest of the body to give it a pleasing look. Symmetry is never sacrificed for size.
Being real is also about being balanced with your lifestyle. It's not about spending crazy hours in the gym or eating boiled chicken and vegetables out of your tupperware container. It's about loving yourself (and the cheesecake) and striving to improve in a holistic manner.

HEALTHY: Fabulous bodies are healthy. What's the point of looking good when you don't feel good? We feel good when we are supremely healthy. However, most people have only a rough idea of what "healthy" is. Is it merely the absence of disease? Is it simply maintaining a healthy weight? Or is it living to a certain age? In this book, I will go deep into explaining how one can progress towards optimal health.

INSPIRATIONAL: Fabulous bodies are inspirational. In life, ultimate fulfilment comes from inspiring and helping people. Once you build a fabulous body, you will naturally inspire people wherever you go. However, you can take this one step further and pursue it actively, which can be done in various ways. For example, you can start donating not just money but time and effort. Don't have a cause? Find one. Ask others to do the same; they may need a small nudge, but they usually oblige. I believe we are all inherently good people who want to help and contribute to our communities.

THE NINE FUNDAMENTAL LAWS FOR BUILDING A FABULOUS BODY

FABULOUS BODY LAW #1:
Less is more: Apply the 80/20 rule to everything you do.

Recently, I read Perry Marshall's amazing book *80/20 Sales and Marketing*, which is based on the premise that the 80/20 rule applies to everything you do.

The 80/20 Rule is the idea that 80 percent of your results come from 20 percent of your effort. It's a principle that can be applied to every facet of your life, and your training is certainly no exception.

For example, out of all the exercises that you do (especially in the gym), just 20 percent of them yield 80 percent of the results you see. Compounded further, only 4 percent of the exercises yield 64 percent of the results. Think about that for a while!

Thousands and thousands of beautiful bodies were sculpted this way in the era before 1959. One such example is Peary Rader, the editor of the famous *Iron Man* magazine. Peary Rader gained almost 100 pounds in two years performing just four exercises and working out twice a week at the most!

This 80/20 principle has worked wonders for me. Over the past few years, I have been cutting my workout time dramatically from around fourteen hours a week to just three to six hours, and I've seen exceptional results!

Shifting your focus to performing those magical 4 percent of exercises in every workout will double your results while freeing up more of your precious time for more meaningful pursuits.

FABULOUS BODY LAW #2:
Progress: Live outside your comfort zone.

If you want to be a better person, you need to progress from old habits to new ones. Similarly, if you want a fitter, better-looking, and healthier body, you need to progress. To do this, you need to go outside of your comfort zone.

Progressing in the weight room (and in your training and life in general) is both a science and an art, and getting the balance right is something that comes from practice. If you do too much too soon, your momentum will break, and you'll become overwhelmed by the sheer effort required to reach your goal. You'll fail, and you'll become fearful.

On the other hand, if you progress slowly and realistically, you will build up a nice momentum in a safe manner. Before you know it, you'll have entered new territories you wouldn't have believed you could achieve.

Let me illustrate this principle with an example. My ultimate goal is to reach 500 pounds in deadlift for ten reps. My previous approach included adding at least 5 kg (about 11 pounds) every week, thinking it would help me reach my goal faster. This was fine in the beginning when my poundage was close to my body weight, but eventually I started compromising my technique to maintain this rate of progress! My knees and lower back started to hurt.

What did I do? As you might have guessed, I dropped the idea of deadlifting altogether, convincing myself it was not a safe exercise. But the real problem was that with this quick approach, I didn't give my body enough time to adapt to the stimulus. If you apply the slow-building yet effective method that I discuss in this book, you'll enjoy every minute of your training By the way, in just a year's time, I was able to deadlift more than 300 pounds for ten reps!

FABULOUS BODY LAW #3:
Go high (or low).

There is a growing body of research that suggests you can get fit in relatively little time. With the recent mega-success of Paleo diets, which mimic the diets of ancient hunter gatherers, researchers are turning to a similar concept in fitness and suggesting a fitness routine similar to the physical activity our ancestors engaged in.

Our genes were built millions of years ago, and if you think about the lifestyle back then, you'll see that our ancestors were either doing short burst of high intensity activities (like saving themselves from wild animals or even hunting them) or low intensity activities for a long period of time, like walking to find shelter or something like that[1]. Forget about doing long, boring moderate-intensity cardio workouts, and perform activities that you are genetically suited for.

FABULOUS BODY LAW #4:
Chew more, eat less, and eat natural foods.

Most of us overeat mainly because we eat too quickly. Many of us also make the mistake of multitasking while we eat—

like watching TV, reading a newspaper, playing with our kids, or even talking on the phone.

Numerous studies have shown that we need to chew our food properly. We need to pay attention to what we are eating and absolutely cherish it. This slow and deliberate way of eating allows for the adequate release of stomach acids, which helps us digest our food. This is known as mindful eating.

The modern approach to meals is the complete opposite of what we should be doing. Eating food used to be a ritual. Family members sat at the dining table and paid attention to eating in the "good old days"! I realize that creating such a perfect meal experience is not always possible for a modern family, but you can at least make sure that you eat slowly. It takes our brain 15 minutes to signal us that we are full. Taking this time to eat results in eating less, and we all know there is strong link between eating less and living longer. But simply eating less is not enough if you want to stay fit and healthy. *What* you eat is also important. Choose food that is as close to its natural state as possible—whole foods over processed foods, saturated fats over vegetable oils, raw milk over pasteurized, grass fed over grain fed meats, and so on.

FABULOUS BODY LAW #5:
Be specific.

One of the most common reason a person drops out of a fitness program is lack of clarity about fitness goals. In one of his fabulous videos, my favorite life coach, Robin Sharma, states that **clarity precedes mastery**.

This idea changed my life. I started contemplating the concept a lot. Do we really know how much muscle we need to gain to have a pleasing look? Do we know the benchmark of how strong should we be? What should be the optimal range of key health indicators, and so on and so forth? At Fabulous Body, I take the idea of clarity very seriously. That's why I have built a whole paradigm with pillars, laws, and criteria surrounding it. During more than a decade of experience in the fitness industry, 90 percent of the people I've worked with simply want to look good and feel good. Fortunately, there is a formula for looking good, which you will read about later in this section.

In Chapter 5, I discuss five **specific** steps to building a fabulous body that will make you so passionate that I promise that over time, working out and eating healthy won't seem like chores to you anymore.

FABULOUS BODY LAW #6:
Get enough Vitamin D.

Consider these facts: More than a billion people worldwide are Vitamin D deficient or insufficient, meaning that their blood levels of this important nutrient are less than 20 mg/dl and levels between 20mg/dl and 29mg/dl respectively[2]. In 2009 researchers from Harvard and the University of Colorado revealed that 70 percent of whites, 90 percent of Hispanics, and 97 percent of blacks in the United States have insufficient blood levels of vitamin D; their study was published in the Archives of Internal Medicine. Near the equator—in South Africa, Saudi Arabia, India, Brazil, and Mexico—estimates are that between 30 percent and upwards of 80 percent of children and adults who have minimum sun exposure are Vitamin D deficient or insufficient[3].

Vitamin D deficiency or insufficiency is the most common medical condition in the world with sometimes devastating, even fatal, consequences. These are not my words but the words of Dr. Michael F Holick, a pioneer of groundbreaking studies in Vitamin D deficiency. Contrary to popular wisdom, he says, Vitamin D isn't just for bone health. It is actually a hormone that plays a central role in metabolism and also in muscle, cardiac, immune, and neurological functions as well in the regulation of inflammation.

Dr. Holick further adds that we have been brainwashed into thinking that exposure to sunlight is bad. This is both unfortunate and untrue. There is no substantiated scientific evidence to suggest that **moderate sun exposure** significantly increases the risk of cancer, even the most deadly form of skin cancer, melanoma.

If you are someone who spends a lot of time indoors behind a desk, has darker skin, lives in a country that hardly gets any sunshine (like Canada), are obese, or are over the age 50, you fall into the high risk category for Vitamin D deficiency. Go out in the sun more often, and get your Vitamin D levels checked today.

FABULOUS BODY LAW #7:
Breathe correctly.

Many people do not understand the impact breathing has on physiological and psychological well-being. Think about how shallow your breath becomes when you are stressed.

Most of us breathe into the upper chest, which is not the best way to breathe because it signals the body that we are under stress even when we are not. In turn, shallow breathing activates the sympathetic nervous system (the fight or flight response).

Instead, practice relaxed diaphragmatic breathing, which is a slow and calm movement of your diaphragm, not your upper chest. Diaphragmatic breathing stimulates the parasympathetic nervous system, which causes the brain to release endorphins which in turn reduces muscle tension and feelings of anxiety.

Deep breathing also oxygenates our blood which keeps our cells in an aerobic state, which then aids in fat loss and increases our energy.

Ideally an adult should take no more than 12-15 breathes in a minute. In order to fully realize the tremendous benefits of deep breathing, aim to consciously take deep breaths throughout the day.

FABULOUS BODY LAW #8:
Optimize sleep.

Optimizing your sleep is an essential element in building a fabulous body. If you don't get enough quality sleep every day, you will never be able to experience optimal health no matter how regularly you exercise or how well you eat, During sleep your body repairs, restores, and rebuilds. Deep sleep triggers key hormones like HGH, which helps you to burn fat and build and repair muscle tissue, whereas lack of sleep can increase your risk of heart disease, diabetes, and stroke. Enough time in the sack can also you help you function well during the day, which can lead to increased productively and happiness.

How much sleep you need to stay healthy and alert depends on your age and may vary. For adults, anywhere between seven and nine hours is recommended.

FABULOUS BODY LAW #9:
Include variety.

As a bodybuilder, I am obsessed with weight training. I love lifting, but I am not in the gym six times a week. I prefer a variety of physical activities. I work out in the gym two to three time a week, and the rest of the week I do HIIT, hatha yoga, swimming, and calisthenics. I am charged about the 10,000 steps daily challenge on my Fitbit device, and I stand and work most of the time. All of this ensures that I am building a well-rounded body that is not only good looking but is functional and healthy.

Life is meant to be enjoyed, and that includes your health and fitness routine. Working out doesn't need to feel like a chore, and variety in your training ensures that it won't. Variety promotes enjoyment and consistency and ensures that you don't get bored.

FBX is not just about weights, cardio, and abs. In fact it's a multifaceted training system that encompasses flexibility and balance, allowing you to use your muscles in all planes of motion as well as use all of your energy systems. This doesn't mean that too much variety is good, though. I perform activities specific to my goals. If I don't like something, I move on, and I usually stick with things I am passionate about. The key is to find things you enjoy doing that are also in alignment with your health and fitness goals.

CHAPTER 4:
CONFESSIONS OF A FABIAN (ONE WHO WORKS OUT USING THE FBX SYSTEM)

I am a physical culturist. I put effort into looking good, but I am not obsessive about it. I don't want a six pack or an overly ripped, shredded look! Even though I know I could achieve these if I wanted them, I am turned off by the obsessive lifestyle and unbalanced approach needed to maintain it.

I am busy. I am a professional who wants to do well in my career and wants to take it to the next level.

Although I wouldn't consider myself a foodie, I'd be lying if I said I didn't love an occasional pizza or burger. I know eating clean and healthy is important but I simply cannot eat only boiled chicken with broccoli all the time, nor can I eat five or six small meals a day or be in the gym that many times per week.

I have a movie to catch, want to spend time with my family, and I have other important commitments. With the FBX Training system, I follow a routine that allows me to get fantastic results in three to six hours a week. The reduced time commitment allows me to be very consistent with my workouts. I progress day after day, month after month, and year after year. I don't lose momentum in a few basic compound movements, and I devote at least 80 percent of my time in the gym to relentlessly progressing in these exercises. Using the multifaceted FBX system, I do a variety of movements and eat a wholesome, homemade, delicious diet.

I do not take boatloads of supplements; instead, I rely on the "fantastic three" to do the job: whey concentrates, omega-3, and multivitamins.

I routinely maintain body fat of around 12 – 15 percent, which gives my six-pack slight visibility. I am happy with the way I look. My friends tell me I look fabulous and they are inspired to do the same, as they think it is achievable.

I am aware that ultimate fulfilment in life comes from inspiring and helping other people and cannot emphasize enough how important it is for me to devote time to giving back not just money but also effort. I don't need to be moved by a cause to start a charity; I am proactive and find a cause. I feel that we are all inherently good people who want to help and contribute to our communities, and I see this in others when they oblige my requests to give back as well.

I am REAL.

I am HEALTHY.

I INSPIRE.

I am FABULOUS!

CHAPTER 5:
FIVE SPECIFIC STEPS FOR BUILDING A FABULOUS BODY

The more specific or explicit the goal, the more precisely performance is regulated."--Edwin Locke, father of modern goal setting.

Consider this analogy: You are a ship, and you have a goal to reach shore in five days. You draw out a map, you check out the weather conditions, and every day you make sure you are on track. Of course there are lot of things that can slow you down, but if you have a clear, specific destination in mind, chances are very high you will reach it. As Zig Ziglar says, "A goal properly set is halfway reached."

On the other hand, if you have no destination and only have a vague idea of where you want to go, you will probably keep moving in circles. Did you know that there are certain neurological processes in the left prefrontal cortex of the brain that acts like a GPS for your goals? Your brain will figure out how to bring the process of achieving your goals into your awareness.

This chapter will teach you to be specific. It will act as a rudder for your ship, making sure you stay on track and keep going in the right direction in order to reach your goal in a timely manner. Let's get started:

Step 1: Determine your sexy weight range and body proportions.

"Too many muscles can get in your way. You have got to have enough to get people interested, but not so much to scare them off." —Steve Reeves (the most admired bodybuilder of the 20th century)

How much is too much? That depends on you. What is your preference? Do you like a lean look, like Brad Pitt in "Fight Club," or do you like more size? How about Chris Hemsworth in "Thor," or Ryan Reynolds in "Green Lantern"?

Dr. Casey Butt has done a brilliant job of finding us a sexy weight range for men that women find attractive.

Sexy Weight Range = Minimum Lean Body Weight: $23 * H^2$ – Maximum Muscular Body Weight: $26 * H^2$

In this equation, height (H) is in meters and weight is in kilograms. You can convert feet and inches to meters here. (www.feettometres.com)

Let's take an example of an individual who is 6 feet tall to illustrate this point better.

His sexy weight range, assuming his body fat is between 9 percent and 14 percent, is 77 kg – 87kg (170 – 192 pounds).

This sexy weight range came from a study by MJ Tovee funded by Newcastle University[4].

In the study, thirty female undergraduates rated color pictures of 50 men in front view. Waist to chest ratio (WCR)—a measure of upper body shape, waist to hip ratio (WHR)—a measure of lower body shape, and BMI were measured for each man. Images were presented in random order with each subject's head and body obscured.

Results showed that individually all three characteristics were contributors to attractiveness. However, WCR was the principal determinant of attractiveness, accounting for 56 percent of the variance, whereas BMI accounted for only 12.7 percent of the additional variance. WHR was not a significant predictor of attractiveness.

What this boils down to is that shape (WCR) is more important for male attractiveness than size, which clearly explains why Steve Reeves was the most admired man of the twentieth century. Even though his weight was well outside the sexy weight range, his shape and especially his WCR (chest: 49/waist: 29=1.68) was exceptional. That's what one should target.

Now there is no doubt that an upper body V-taper, broad shoulders, and a big chest that tapers down to a narrow waist is attractive to the opposite sex.

This effect can also be linked back to the **golden ratio** and da Vinci's **Vitruvian Man.** Let's discuss them briefly:

In mathematics, two quantities are in the **golden ratio** if their ratio is the same as the ratio of their sum to the larger of the two quantities. The figure below illustrates this geometric relationship:

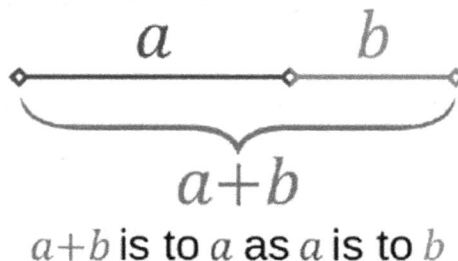

$$a \qquad\qquad b$$

$$a+b$$

$a+b$ is to a as a is to b

Where b is 1 unit long, and a is 1.618 unit long and algebraically they can be explained as: a+b/a = a/b =(GR)= **1.6180**

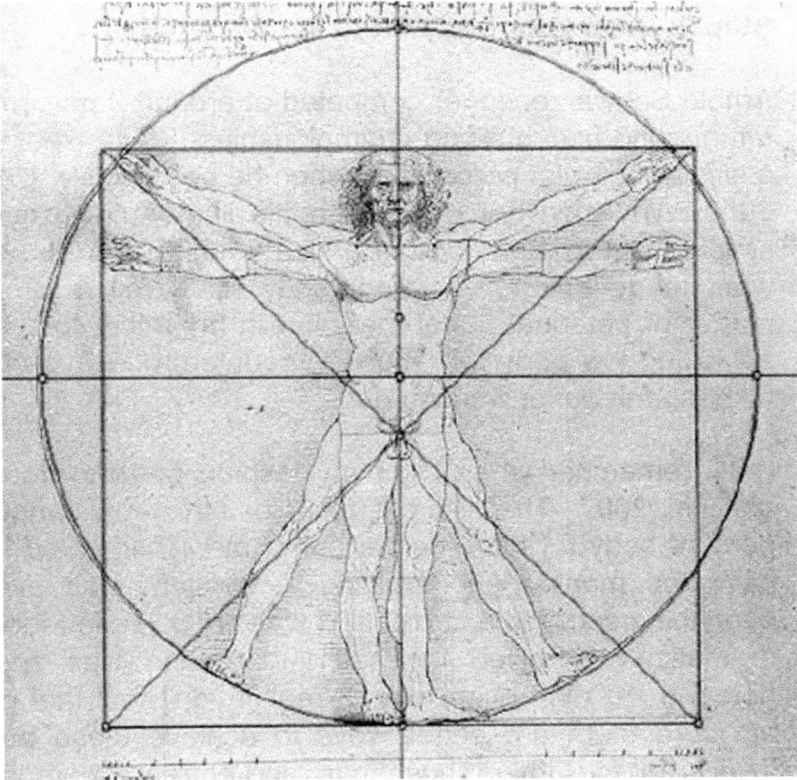

Vitruvian Man is perhaps Leonardo da Vinci's most famous illustration and is based on the work of the architect Vitruvius. The illustration in the picture below reflects the golden ratio and Leonardo's keen interest in proportions. This picture also represents da Vinci's attempt to relate man to nature—he firmly believed that the workings of the human body are analogous to the workings of the universe.

While further discussion on this topic is beyond the scope of this book, the fact is that **a shoulder width approximately 1.6 times the width of your waist will make you look the**

best, and the fastest way to reach this goal is to make sure your waist is as small as it can get. This brings us to the next step.

Step 2: Drop your body fat to 9 – 14 percent.

Arnold Schwarzenegger competed at around 9 percent body fat in world bodybuilding championships. Steve Reeves had a similar body fat percentage when he became Mr. Universe 1950. Why then do average people like you and me, who simply want to look good in a slim fit shirt or on the beach, want to go below 9 percent body fat? Well, again it's a matter of personal preference, but in my mind, focusing on achieving low body fat ranges is counterproductive and can take the fun out of working out.

I still remember when I got my fashion portfolio done way back in 2007. The effort it took to achieve a range of 7 percent body fat took the life out of me. Thank God I didn't have too many responsibilities at the time, but even so, everything came to a standstill. I was eating boiled food, had dramatically reduced my salt intake, and was spending hours in the gym every day. It really didn't feel that good. I am sure there are better ways to achieve these body fat levels, but for fathers, husbands, and entrepreneurs like you and me, devoting enormous amounts of energy and time just to look extra ripped is futile, and in most cases unnecessary.

I honestly think staying within the 12 – 15 percent body fat range is ideal for most of us. Fabulous Body is about being **real** with your lifestyle, and aiming for low single-digit body fat is overwhelming and almost like a full-time job. Up to 15 percent gives a slight visibility of six-pack abs, and it's good enough for most of us.

I have been maintaining the 12 – 15 percent range for quite some time now, and I've hardly had to give up any of my favorite foods. Life is meant to be enjoyed, and building a fabulous body is about balance, both in the gym and outside. In the end, I strongly feel your fitness and health goals should enhance your life, not consume it.

Step 3: Optimize your key health indicators.

My most often used statement on my blog, fabulousbody.com, is: *What's the point of looking good when you don't feel good*?

Being a physical culturist is fine; after all, looking good is somewhat tied to self-esteem and confidence, but being obsessed about it can create many problems. One of these problems is a major image disorder, which further leads to an obsessive lifestyle that may include extreme diets, long hours in the gym every day, very high proteins diets, excessive use of supplements, or even drugs and steroid use. You may attract a few stares, but at what cost? Building a fabulous body is all about building a body that not only looks good, but is also optimally healthy and functional.

So let's look at a few important numbers that can determine overall how **healthy** we actually are. There are a few more health indicators besides the ones discussed below, but these three are usually of significant importance: fasting insulin, cholesterol, and resting heart rate.

Fasting Insulin

Insulin is a hormone released by the beta cells of your pancreas. It helps sugar move from your blood to your cells where it can be used for energy or stored as glycogen in liver and muscles. If you eat too many carbs (especially in the form of simple sugars like cakes and pastries) too often, more insulin is released to combat that extra sugar. Over time, your cells become insensitive to the excess insulin, which ultimately leads to insulin sensitivity.

The higher your insulin levels, the worse your insulin resistance. Elevated fasting insulin is the single greatest marker for assessing a person's risk for cardiovascular disease and diabetes[5,6].
Your fasting insulin levels can be determined by a blood test. A normal range should be less than 5, ideally less than 3. If your insulin is above 5, aim to reduce your sugar intake to bring it down.

Cholesterol

Cholesterol is a soft, white waxy substance found in every cell in your body. It's used to produce cell membranes, Vitamin D, hormones, etc. More than 25 percent of the cholesterol in your body is found in your brain.

It's a myth that cholesterol is evil, but it's so much ingrained in people's mind that it is bad that they will do anything to lower cholesterol levels to below 200 mg/dl. However, the fact remains that total cholesterol is a poor indicator of risk for heart disease; rather, the following two ratios are much better indicators[7].

HDL/Total Cholesterol: Ideally this ratio should exceed 24 percent. Below 10 percent predicts an increased risk for heart disease.

Triglycerides/HDL ratio: This ratio should be less than 2[8,9].

Resting heart rate (RHR)

RHR is the heart rate of a person at rest. For an average person, it varies from 70 – 80 beats per minute. Together, the heart rate and the stroke volume (amount of blood pumped out with each contraction of a ventricle) make up the overall performance of the heart. A high RHR indicates that your heart is working harder to pump oxygenated blood throughout your body, whereas a low RHR indicates that you are fit, as your heart is able to pump more forcefully and push more blood with every beat.

Ideally your RHR should be less than 65 BPM. The lower the better. Trained athletes have RHRs somewhere in the 40s and 50s! There have been various studies published that clearly suggest a direct link between how many times your heart beats per minute and the risk of heart disease[10]. One study even claims that people with low resting heart rates cut their risk of diabetes in half[11].

Here's how you can manually monitor your heart rate: It's best to take this measurement yourself as soon as you wake up in the morning and before you get out of bed. Start a stop watch and gently press the inside of your wrist with two fingers. Remember the touch should be gentle, and the reading should be taken as soon as you wake up. Remain calm and take the reading a few times for accuracy.

Step 4: Functional Fitness: Build a body capable of doing real-life activities effectively.

Bodybuilders are guilty of performing isolated exercises mainly using machines that emphasize only one plane of motion—the sagittal plane. This causes muscle imbalances, and your muscles become prone to injury.

In real life, our muscles are used to working in all three planes of motion: sagittal, frontal, and transverse. Yes, there are three planes of motions.

Sagittal plane is forward or backward. Most gym movements, like lat pulldown, bench press, and biceps curl are in this plane of motion.

Frontal plane is side to side. Movements like lateral raise, side lunges, and side shuffling are in this plane.

Transverse plane is rotational. Swinging a golf club is an example of moving in the transverse plane.

THREE PLANES OF MOTION

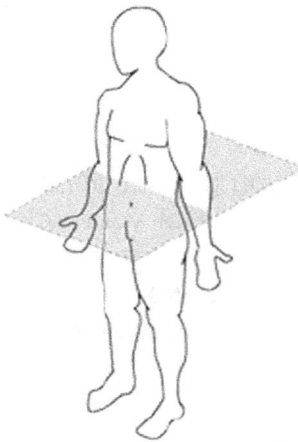 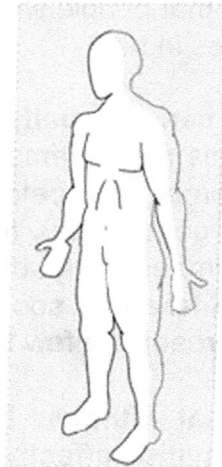 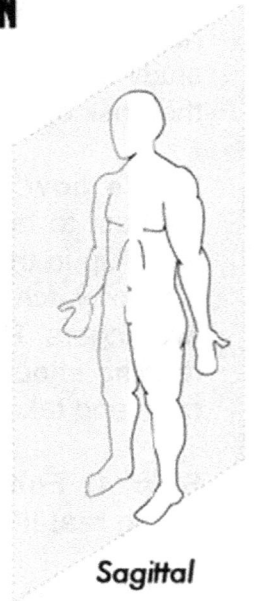

Transverse   Frontal   Sagittal

As you must have figured, most of us perform movements in the sagittal plane, hence it becomes imperative to include movements in the frontal and transverse planes as well. Ideally this can be achieved by using functional whole-body exercises involving multiple planes of motion and multiple joints, which mimics real-life activities. Think squat, deadlift, wood chop, and medicine ball side throw (rotational exercises) to name a few.

Once you start doing FBX workouts, where most of the exercises are functional and mainly involve the whole body, you will build real-life functional strength. You will be able to swim long enough and carry your wife's shopping bags and your infant kid up 10 floors when the elevator is not working, making it look really easy. Weekend warriors, I know how much you love your sport. You will be able to play any sport you like with relative ease. And, you will be able to save yourself from a ferocious street dog should the situation arise!

Step 5: Become strong.

Strength is celebrated. Over the centuries, men have played the role of protector, defender, and warrior. Strength is one of the main things that separates a man from women. DUH!

In these modern times with all the technological advances, men are often required to sit behind a desk all day, but even then there is something primal in us that makes us want to become a stronger version of ourselves—to take care of ourselves and our families if need be, to push back if being pushed, etc. It's my belief that strength is an essential virtue for every man to have.

In my experience, the strength that we build in the weight room does transcend into other forms of strength (strength of character, strength of spirit, etc.), but that's a topic for some other day. For now, let's focus on the benchmarks of physical strength.

How strong should be a man be?

For starters, if you can pull your bodyweight a few times over and can perform dips for at least 5 – 8 reps, you are considered strong. (You'd be surprised to know that the majority of men are not able to perform these simple feats.)

In the gym fraternity, strength is measured with four exercises:

1. Squats
2. Deadlifts
3. Bench press
4. Overhead press

The following numbers are guidelines, not definitive numbers. Reaching these numbers can take years and roughly correspond to reaching your genetic potential (the amount of muscle your body is able to gain naturally).

squats: 2 * bodyweight

deadlift: 2.5 * bodyweight

bench press: 1.5 * bodyweight

overhead press: 1 * bodyweight

For a 180-pound man, these number corresponds to:

squats: 360 pounds

deadlift: 450 pounds

bench press: 270 pounds

overhead press: 180 pounds

Also note that these numbers corresponds to your 1 Rep Max.

CHAPTER 6:
FOUR BULLETPROOF MINDSET PRINCIPLES FOR SUREFIRE RESULTS

Did you know that the quickest way to change your life—and your body—is to change your mind? Successful people have a unique mindset when it comes to the way they view life. Developing a mindset is about developing habits. You must have heard the following quote a million times by now:

We are what we repeatedly do. Excellence, then, is not an act but a habit. -- **Aristotle**

Our mind is only 10 percent conscious, which means that 90 percent of our thought processes are subconscious. We act according to the conditioning of our subconscious mind. Therefore, we need to train our subconscious to assist us in our daily lives to achieve the results we desire.

We are conditioned to wake up in the morning and brush our teeth, take a shower, and follow our routine, right? It makes sense, therefore, that we can also condition ourselves to eat a healthy diet or follow a simple weight training routine day after day, month after month, and year after year. Why can't we build these habits over time so that a healthy lifestyle comes naturally to us?

You may have heard a lot of buzz about the so-called 21-day rule, but the truth is that it takes 66 days to build a new habit[12]. Why can't we dedicate 66 days of our lives to building the most important habit of all—healthy living—and build our dream physique in the process? The question always remains: **How badly do we want it?**

Working out, eating at least 500 grams of raw vegetables every day, and consuming 1.4 – 2.0 grams per kg of bodyweight of protein is so ingrained in me that I don't have to plan it. It comes as naturally to me as breathing does because I took the time to build the habit. That's all you have to do; start small and build it over time.

Let me tell you a secret: The first steps are the most difficult ones, and after that it gets significantly easier. There are three phases we go through when we try to achieve a goal: the beginning, the middle, and the end. As Robin Sharma puts it, the beginning is the toughest, it's messy in the middle, but it's beautiful at the end.

The beginning of most things can be difficult. It's like pushing a stationary train, and it can feel like an impossible feat in those early days. However, when you understand that doing that thing is important (whether it's joining a gym, opening a business, or getting up early in the morning), you use your willpower and push through it. Again, the key is to start small.

As James Clear says in his free guide, *Transform Your Habits*:

"It's incredibly easy to get caught up in the desire to make massive changes in your life. We watch incredible weight loss transformations and think that we need to lose 30 pounds in the next 4 weeks. We see elite athletes on TV and wish that we could run faster and jump higher tomorrow. We want to earn more, do more and be more... right now. I've felt those things, so I get it. Although I applaud this enthusiasm, it's important to keep in mind that lasting

*change is a product of daily habits, not once-in-a-lifetime transformations. If you want to start a new habit and begin living healthier and happier, I cannot emphasize this enough: **start small**. In the words of Leo Babauta, "Make it so easy that you can't say no."*

How small should you start? Stanford professor B.J. Fogg suggests that people who want to start flossing begin by flossing only one tooth. Just one. Performance doesn't matter in the beginning. What matters is becoming the type of person who always sticks to your new habit, no matter how small or insignificant it seems. You can build up to the level of performance that you want once your behavior becomes consistent. If you've become lazy and want to start a fitness regimen, you can start by doing one push-up or taking the stairs and then build it up over time."

Life is all about the accumulation of these small successes. Over time, they compound until you eventually reach true success. **I love this quote by soccer sensation Lionel Messi: "*I start early, and I stay late, day after day after day, year after year. It took me 17 years and 114 days to become an overnight success.*"**

Always think about how far you have come rather than how far you have left to go. You'll find that when you start thinking this way, a whole new world opens up for you! Don't believe me? Try it! What do you have to lose?

Here are four key mindset principles that will guide you through. Adopting them will pretty much guarantee your success:

1. **Think long term.** When you're trying to build the body that you want, nothing can override the need for time. If you ask me how much time it takes to build a lean, attractive, healthy physique, I'll tell you that it depends. So many things

go into it—your training history, the intensity of your workouts, how disciplined you are with your nutrition, how much rest and sleep you are getting every day, genetics, and most of all how motivated you are every day to achieve your goals.

Motivation needs constant refueling. You need to build momentum, and you need to be inspired by a long-term vision. Imagine an avalanche; once it gets rolling, there is no stopping it.

If you are truly inspired to do something, you are in it for the long haul. Your mind will view any problems or setbacks as temporary, and you'll have a clear and specific vision of where you want yourself to be after a set period of time. You'll have a clear, step-by-step plan written down to achieve your goal.

Once you have a clear vision of what you want to achieve, the next step is to build a routine. **A routine is a collection of certain strong habits that will propel you effortlessly towards your dream physique.**

In today's society, people seem to live by the following motto: I want it all, and I want it now, even if it means resorting to pills, tablets, or injections to achieve it.

It is true that we often need to pay a price to look good and feel good. If it was easy and could be achieved in just few months, everyone would already be there. If you look around, it's actually the opposite. It might sound trite, but **it's crucial to keep in mind that everything worth achieving is worth working hard for.**

This might not be what you want to hear, but no special workout, diet, or supplement can override the need for time. I have been training for more than a decade now. I've made tons of mistakes along the way, but I never lost hope, and I eventually found better and smarter ways to build my body through sheer perseverance.

So how long will it take to build the body of your dreams? If you work hard and follow the FBX (Fabulous Body) system of training explained in this book, I think you can dramatically alter your physique in about six months to one year. Too long? That amount of time will pass anyway.

If you try a program that promises extreme results, you might notice some quick improvements, but they will go away just as quickly. The beauty lies in the journey, not the destination. Cherish it, enjoy it, struggle with it, and before you know it, success will be yours!

2. **Desire: You have to want it, and you have to want it badly—really badly**! Your burning desire is directly proportional to how soon you will achieve success. You need to have sufficient reasons for doing something. If you don't spend enough time analyzing your "why," just a few small obstacles will be enough to knock you off track.

The buck stops with you. You alone are responsible for your results. Are you prepared to give it your best shot? Do you plan to reach your goals no matter what comes up along the way?**If your answer is a resounding "yes," your quest to achieve a lean, fit, healthy physique is almost guaranteed!**

At times, you'll want to give up. Sometimes you might work very hard and feel like nothing is happening. When you're feeling like this, your solid reason—your "why"—will keep you going. You will keep eating healthy food instead of a pizza because you know the former will bring you closer to your most coveted goal. Your goal is dear to you, and you know that when you achieve it, you will feel a sense of pride and accomplishment. Isn't that what life is all about?

3. **Instinct and guts: Listen to your gut. It doesn't lie to you.** There is so much information out there, but most of it is bad information. You need to trust someone. You bought this book because somehow you felt that I could be trusted.

You cannot rely on too many coaches or different websites. You need to find someone you can trust, someone you like, and someone you think is telling the truth. There are a lot of scammers out there who simply want your money. They don't care about you; they just want your money. Nevertheless, certain individuals really do care about you and are in it for the long haul. Your instincts will tell you the truth!

I almost gave up after ten years of failing miserably to gain muscles on my thin frame. Why? I was being guided by conventional wisdom. I trusted it blindly. I did what everyone was doing and ended up looking like them—weak, fat and flabby. In my heart, I knew I needed to dig deeper.

Steve Reeves gave me that hope. When I read about him, I could tell instantly that he wanted to help people. When I read about Stuart McRoberts, John McCullum, Dr. Mercola, and Ori Hofmekler, I knew these individuals were independent researchers who would share the truth. I trusted them and applied their concepts, choosing only specific things that resonated with me, and I got fantastic results. That's really all you need to do! If you can pick one or two ideas from this book and from my website fabulousbody.com that resonate with you perfectly and get you results, I will be delighted.

4. **Be committed.** If you want spectacular results, you need to truly commit from the bottom of your heart no matter what, even if it takes longer than you anticipate. You need to know that it's about the journey and that anything that is worth achieving is not easy (although my book will simplify things

for you)! Only you can commit yourself. No one else can do it for you.

The word "mediocre" is derived from the Latin *mediocris*, which means "halfway up a mountain." This time, you need to fully commit yourself to reaching the top of the mountain no matter what.

CHAPTER 7:
THE REAL SCIENCE OF FAT LOSS: THREE KEY PRINCIPLES

You are not fat; you have fat. Fat doesn't define you! I always tell my clients that amount of body fat is directly proportional to their lifestyle.

Everyone's body fat level has a certain lifestyle attached to it.

Our goal is to be below 15 percent and ideally at 12 percent. Let's look at three key fat loss principles that will melt fat like butter.

Fat loss principle number #1: You must eat 15 to 20 percent less than your total daily energy expenditure (TDEE) in order to lose weight.

Losing weight is a simple equation of calories in versus calories out. Here is the easiest way to understand energy balance:

Energy Balance = Energy Intake – Energy Expenditure

Energy intake encompasses everything you put into your mouth.

Energy expenditure consists of several factors, including resting metabolic rate (RMR), caloric cost of activity, and the thermic effect of food (TEF). The balance of intake versus output is a critical starting point in weight gain or loss.

There are several formulas you can use to calculate the total number of calories you burn in a day as you will see in Section 2.

If you have a SURPLUS of calories (positive energy balance) where the intake exceeds the expenditure, you gain weight.

If you have a DEFICIT of calories (negative energy balance) where the intake is less than expenditure, you lose weight.

Does that sound simple enough? This is actually just a starting principle, but it's an important one nevertheless.

The type of calories you consume are the next consideration. You need to make sure that the calories you eat come from food that is nutrient-dense rather than typical fast food. We will discuss the type of calories you should eat in more detail in the nutrition section.

Fat loss principle #2: A combination of HIIT and weight training is necessary to achieve maximum fat loss.

Consider this: Trapp, et. al., conducted a study in which young women performed HIIT for 15 weeks with three 20-minute sessions per week. HIIT consisted of an 8-second sprint followed by 12 seconds of low intensity cycling, repeated for 20 minutes. Another group of women carried out an aerobic cycling protocol for 40 minutes each session. Results showed that women in the HIIT group lost 2.5 kg of subcutaneous fat, whereas no change occurred with steady state aerobic exercise. Fat loss accruing through 15 weeks of HIIT was attained with 50 percent less exercise time and a similar energy expenditure to that of steady state exercise[13].

In addition to HIIT, FBX's bed rock activity is weight training three times a week. With weights, you build muscles, and muscles burn more fat. We know muscles are catabolically more active tissues than fat, meaning they need more energy to survive. So if one gains 10 pounds of muscles, he or she will burn roughly 50 to 70 calories more per day without even moving. Isn't that awesome? Besides this, weight training has an EPOC effect and can boost your metabolism for up to 16 hours (sometimes more depending on the intensity of your workouts). This added advantage of elevated metabolism results in more calorie burn without doing anything[14]!

Fat loss principle #3: Intermittent fasting is an effective way to lose fat.

Intermittent fasting typically means a smaller eating window and eating fewer meals than a person would normally eat in a day. There are various ways in which one can practice intermittent fasting. One can eat normally for five days and then cut food intake by around 25 percent over the weekend. Or another way is to skip breakfast and fast until lunch.
With intermittent fasting, people end up eating fewer calories overall than they would when they eat say 3 – 5 meals in a day and therefore it can help in reducing your total caloric intake, which in turn can be beneficial to heart health and chronic disease prevention[15,16,17,18].

Consider another study in the *British Medical Journal* in which sixteen obese adults were given an energy restricted diet for a period of eight weeks randomized into two treatment arms (high meal frequency = three meals + three snacks/day or low meal frequency= three meals/day). It was concluded that increased meal frequency does not promote greater body weight loss[19].

In the nutrition section, I discuss my more than a year experience with intermittent fasting and my weekly diet plan using this concept.

CHAPTER 8:
THE REAL SCIENCE OF MUSCLE BUILDING: THREE KEY PRINCIPLES

Our main goal is to get bigger muscles. Don't worry, not the puffy bodybuilder kind, but rock hard, lean muscles. We established in Chapter 5 that being in your sexy weight range will make you look dramatically better than majority of the guys out there assuming your body fat is in the 9 to 14 percent range. Yes, this is all that is needed, and if you do it the Fabulous Body way, you will be headed towards optimal health.

I am a student of the science behind real muscle building, and in this chapter I will unlock for you the true principles of how to build muscles effectively.

Muscle growth principle number #1: Muscular overload

"Your strength is directly proportional to the size of your muscles." Paste this statement somewhere where you will see it every day. This statement is the universal truth, and if someone is telling you otherwise, they are simply lying or are not aware of the mechanisms of muscle growth.

Yes there are some minor exceptions to this fact—bone structure, muscle attachments, and neural factors also play a role in performing "feats of strength." Note that performance strength is different from the strength I am talking about, though. Performance strength is built via performing very low reps (1 – 5) and multiple sets (5 – 6). It is based on neural factors and is mainly used by powerlifters and other performance strength athletes whose main goal is not size but simply pure brute strength!

The strength that I am talking about is what happens through **progressive weight lifting done with low to moderate reps.** In the FBX routines discussed in the training section, you will read that I usually advocate a two rep range, i.e. 5 – 7 for the growth phase and 8 – 10 for the cut phase.

There are a few reasons for the variation in rep range. For this we need to briefly understand the prime factors that trigger muscle growth: **muscular tension** and **metabolic stress**.

Muscular tension

The best way to create muscular tension is to perform a set of low to moderate rep range (3 – 7) with full range of motion. Over time, your muscles will adapt to the muscular tension a particular weight is generating, so you will need to progressively overload, that is, increase the weight while maintaining the low to moderate rep range. **The bottom line is that heavier weights equal greater tension.**

Besides creating tension in your muscles through progressive overload, numerous studies support an anabolic role of exercise-induced metabolic stress[20,21,22], **although it's important to note** that metabolic stress does not seem to be an essential component of muscular growth[23].

Metabolic stress

Metabolic stress manifests as a result of exercise that relies on anaerobic glycolysis for ATP production, which results in the subsequent buildup of metabolites such as lactate, hydrogen ions, inorganic phosphates, creatine, and others[24,25]. Buildup of these metabolites has been shown to impact anabolic processes[26]. Metabolic stress is associated with pump training and fills up the fluid part of the muscle cell.

In the end, remember this: Pump training (muscular fatigue) through moderate rep ranges of 8 – 12 induces more metabolic stress than muscular tension, and I believe it is only icing on the cake.

Getting a pump is easy, but getting stronger in key compound lifts is tough work!
To better grasp this concept, we will briefly discuss the concept of myofibrillar and sacroplasmic hypertrophy in the training section.

Muscle growth principle number #2: Sleep

No matter how good your training program or your nutrition is, if you don't sleep enough, you are not giving your body enough time to recover. During recovery the body replaces, repairs, and rebuilds tissue (including muscle tissue).

When you sleep, large amounts of growth hormones are released[27]. Human growth hormone (HGH), a hormone, released by the pituitary gland, is vital for physical strength, health, and longevity. HGH is often called the "fountain of youth" as it helps in cell regeneration and slows down the aging process. It also helps build muscles and burn fat[28,29].

So what is the ideal amount of sleep? I would suggest 7 – 9 hours of uninterrupted sleep per night. Make it a habit to practice strong before-bed rituals that you can follow every day for a good quality, uninterrupted sleep.

Try to commit to a set bedtime every day. Turn off your TV and other electronic devices (this may be tough for many of us to do, so just try to minimize use) at least an hour or so before going to bed. Make sure your room is dark (even a little bit of light can interfere with your melatonin levels and prevent you from falling to sleep). If these things do not help, try taking a bath and/or meditating.

Muscle growth and enough quality sleep go hand in hand; therefore making sleep a priority will ensure that you grow.

Muscle growth principle number #3: Nutrition

If you want to build a house (build muscles) then you need materials. If you want to have muscles, you have to feed them, plain and simple. **To gain lean muscles you need to eat more calories than your TDEE (15 – 20 percent). If you don't, your muscles won't grow!**

Having said that, the calories need to come from good quality and a variety of healthy foods. Now, protein as we know, is *the* word in the bodybuilding circuit, and it is for a reason. Yes, a high protein diet is the key. There are studies that confirm that you need at least 1.4 - 2 grams/kilogram of bodyweight in protein[30,31,32]. However, going beyond 2 grams/kilogram of bodyweight shows no significant increase in muscle growth[33].

OK, we got the protein. What next? Most bodybuilders and weight trainers I know only think about protein and neglect other nutrients in their diet. Eating protein is simply part of the whole story. Muscle building is a complex process, and it requires other nutrients in adequate amounts every day. These nutrients are complex carbohydrates, healthy fats (including omega-3), vitamins, minerals and phytonutrients. More on this in the nutrition section.

Muscle building is therefore the art and science of applying the core principles of getting stronger, maximizing sleep and getting proper nutrition over a period of months and years. When you do this, you will be rewarded with more muscles in the process.

SECTION 2: TRAINING

CHAPTER 9:
FBX: INTRODUCING THE FABULOUS BODY TRAINING SYSTEM

Now, let's move from understanding principles to putting those principles into action. This is where the rubber meets the road. Once we have the right mindset, once we know exactly what we want, the doing part becomes relatively easy.

With the recent mega-success of paleo diets, which mimic the diets of ancient hunter-gatherers, research also suggests that a fitness routine similar to the activities our ancestors routinely performed is most effective. In general, hunter-gatherers were lean and probably almost never obese.

James H. O' Keefe's comprehensive research into the lifestyle of hunter-gatherers describes their lifestyle as follows[34]:

- *A large amount of light to moderate activity, such as walking. Most estimates indicate that hunter-gatherers covered an average daily distance in the range of 6 – 16 km (3.7 – 10 miles).*

- *Hard days, resulting in expenditures of at least 800 – 1200 kcal, were typically followed by easier days.*

- *Life in the wild often called for intermittent bursts of moderate to high level intensity exercise (hunting and stalking animals, shelter construction, carrying 20 –*

30 kg of meat back to camp, etc.) with intervening periods of rest and recovery.

☐ *Their routines promoted aerobic endurance, flexibility, and strength, thereby providing them with multifaceted fitness. This varied pattern of movement would have also conferred resiliency and reduced the likelihood of injury, allowing them to hunt and forage without major interruptions.*

☐ *Virtually all of the exercise was done outdoors in the natural world. Outdoor activities helps maintain ultraviolet-stimulated Vitamin D synthesis.*

☐ *Ample rest, relaxation, and sleep were generally available to ensure complete recovery after strenuous exertion.*

In addition to these guidelines on hunter-gatherers, which give us a good idea of what kind of training protocol to follow, let's look at what ACSM (American College of Sports Medicine) suggests for a healthy adult between 14 and 65 years of age.

The official ACSM guidelines for exercise are 30 minutes of low to moderate activity each day. However, many people have misconstrued these guidelines and count a "general stroll" as a form of exercise.

ACSM (American College of Sports Medicine) clears up the confusion with these specific guidelines[35]:

Cardiorespiratory Exercise

☐ *Adults should get at least 150 minutes of moderate-intensity exercise per week.*

☐ *Exercise recommendations can be met through 30 – 60 minutes of moderate-intensity exercise five days* *per week **or 20 – 60 minutes of vigorous-intensity exercise three days per week.***

☐ *One continuous session and multiple shorter sessions of at least 10 minutes are both acceptable to accumulate the desired amount of daily exercise.*

☐ *Gradual progression of exercise time, frequency, and intensity is recommended for best adherence and least risk of injury.*

☐ *People unable to meet these minimums can still benefit from some activity.*

Resistance Exercise

☐ *Adults should train each major muscle group two or three days each week using a variety of exercises and equipment.*

☐ *Very light or light intensity is best for older persons or previously sedentary adults starting exercise.*

☐ *Two to four sets of each exercise will help adults improve strength and power.*

☐ *For each exercise, 8 – 12 repetitions improves strength and power, 10 – 15 repetitions improves strength in middle age and older persons starting exercise, and 15 – 20 repetitions improves muscular endurance.*

☐ *Adults should wait at least 48 hours between resistance training sessions.*

Flexibility Exercise

☐ *Adults should do flexibility exercises at least two or three days each week to improve range of motion.*

☐ *Each stretch should be held for 10 – 30 seconds to the point of tightness or slight discomfort.*

☐ *Repeat each stretch two to four times for a total of 60 seconds per stretch.*

☐ *Static, dynamic, ballistic, and PNF stretches are all effective.*

☐ *Flexibility exercise is most effective when the muscle is warm. Try light aerobic activity or a hot bath to warm the muscles before stretching.*

Neuromotor Exercise

☐ *Neuromotor exercise (sometimes called "functional fitness training") is recommended for two or three days per week.*

☐ *Exercises should involve motor skills (balance, agility, coordination, and gait), proprioceptive exercise training, and multifaceted activities, such as tai ji and yoga, to improve physical function and prevent falls in older adults.*

☐ *Twenty to thirty minutes per day is appropriate for neuromotor exercise.*

THE FBX TRAINING SYSTEM

Recall Fabulous Body Law # 9: Include Variety. Variety is the spice of life, and that includes your workout. You need cardio fitness, strength, flexibility, balance, and agility. All in all, you need a multifaceted fitness system that not only makes you look good but also functional and optimally healthy. The whole idea here is to optimize your gene expression, and you don't need more than three to six hours of exercise per week to do this.

After analyzing the above data (lifestyle of hunter-gatherers and ACSM guidelines) and combining it with principles and wisdom from the "Golden Age of Bodybuilding," I have created a system that will give you fabulous results in minimal time.

FBX workout routines are hybrid between full body and conventional spilt routines. You only need to work out three times a week (sometimes even two times will be enough) using mainly compound exercises with minimal use of isolated exercises.

There are four components to the FBX training system:

1. Weight training (2 – 3 times a week)
2. HIIT (2 – 4 sessions, 20 minutes each)
3. 10,000 daily steps (incorporating more walking and standing in your daily lifestyle)
4. Flexibility and neuromotor activities

FBX TRAINING SYSTEM

ACTIVITY	TIME DEVOTED (HOURS PER WEEK)	INTENSITY	FREQUENCY (TIMES PER WEEK)	PLACE
WEIGHT TRAINING	2 – 4 HOURS	MODERATE/ HIGH	2 – 3	GYM/HOME GYM
HIIT	40 MINUTES – 1.5 HOURS	LOW / HIGH	2 – 4	HOME/GYM
10,000 DAILY STEPS	N/A	LOW	N/A	N/A

ACTIVITY	TIME DEVOTED (HOURS PER WEEK)	INTENSITY	FREQUENCY (TIMES PER WEEK)	PLACE
FLEXIBILITY AND NEUROMOTOR ACTIVITY/ PROTOCOL	1 – 1.5 HOURS	LOW / MODERATE	2 – 3	HOME/GYM

Let's discuss each of these components in more detail.

Weight Training

How spilt routines and training five to six times a week came into vogue

The Canadian bodybuilder Joe Weider, who is often referred to as the father of modern bodybuilding, introduced high volume training —spilt routines i.e. working out **more** than three times a week using isolated exercises for every body part, in the late 1950s.

Great physiques had already been produced (like those of Grimek, Ross, Stephan, Reeves, Eiferman, etc.), **so it is not clear whether high volume training really added anything**.

Joe was always looking for a marketing angle to be new and different from his competition, so he may have promoted high volume spilt routine training as a marketing ploy to be different and not because it provided anything of real value.

Steroids were introduced in 1959, and after that there was no looking back. Bodybuilders could stay in the gym three to four hours a day, six times a week and really focus on specializing each body part and training their muscles from every angle. This allowed them to build a perfectly defined, chiseled physique, which surely gave them that edge over their competitors.

This whole spilt routine thing was further amplified by bodybuilding judges, who started to focus more on an extra-ripped look, more size, and more definition, etc. Awards were given for "best legs," or "best pectorals" and not for "best physique."

The pleasing aspect of a physique was simply replaced by size. "The bigger the better," judges said.

Then the supplement companies took advantage of this trend and started marketing their products by hiring the champion bodybuilders to promote supplements to the masses! Again, "the more the better."

Isn't it a nice coincidence that for most people working out today, the workout culture began with Arnold Schwarzenegger! My bodybuilding story started after I was motivated by Arnold's documentary, "Pumping Iron." That was during the 1970s era of bodybuilding when steroid use was very common in the bodybuilding circuit.

Do you ever ponder why the muscle and fitness magazines conveniently leave out the Golden Era of bodybuilding—the 1940s and 1950s—when there was no supplement use (other than Weider/Hoffman protein shakes—not sure of the quality though) Do you wonder how, in those earlier days, people worked out two to three times a week with full body routines and looked like this:

In the 1940s and 1950s, bodybuilders looked pleasing and

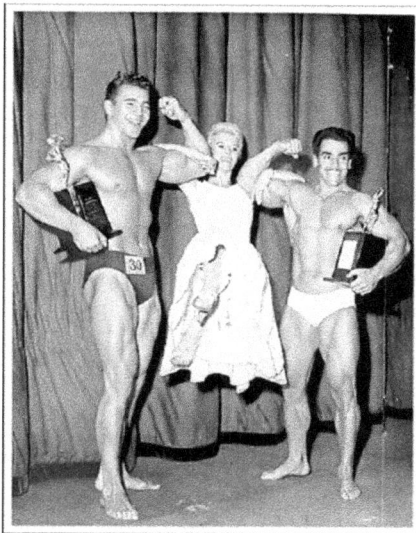

better than bodybuilders you find these days; the majority of us would agree on that point. Then isn't it common sense to train like someone you want to look like? Remember they only worked out three times a week maximum!

As for Arnold, he started using spilt routines only after having built sufficient mass using full body routines three times a week! Why, then, do people like you and me with average genetics want to use spilt routines when most of us have not even built sufficient mass?

I followed modern conventional training (spilt routines) for a decade, and I failed terribly. Most of my gains have come only in the past few years after I started following a more abbreviated training system.

Six Benefits of Working Out Three Times a Week Instead of Five or Six

1. **Training three times a week with FBX workouts will leave you ample time to recover.**

There are two components to training: stimulating the muscular system, *which happens in the gym*, and being able to recover, *which happens outside the gym*. I wrote this book mainly for individuals like you and me who have average genetics, who are pressed for time, who have occasional late nights out, and who have a life outside of training.

Recovery, therefore, needs to be a priority, and that means getting enough sleep, good nutrition, and less stress overall with more rest in general.

Well, you may tell me that your muscles are recovering even after working out six times a week (very rare unless you have exceptional genetics or are on drugs), but what about your nervous system? Oh yes, your nerves also get a workout every time you train! Therefore, if your nervous system is not recovering from your training, you're not maximizing your progress[36].

Your workouts will be stale and performed with no enthusiasm, and your intensity levels will drastically drop!

2. **FBX workouts are practical.**

Consider this scenario: Keith has been performing a single-body part spilt and goes to the gym first thing in the morning to work out for only 45 minutes with weights. He is supercharged with this routine. For how long? Maybe a week or two. What if one day his baby falls sick and he is unable to sleep properly through the night? He is planning to train his legs the next day, and he doesn't want to miss it. He is having doubts about whether he will be able to squat 250 pounds the next morning. The same moment his personal trainer calls him and wants to hear no excuse. Keith gives in, probably gulps down a pre-workout drink (recommended only by his trainer) and gets through a gruesome leg workout.

Or let's assume that Keith is still not married. Well, don't tell me he won't be up until 2:00 am watching bad TV or at a late night get-together with friends. Okay, forget about distractions. What if he simply doesn't feel like going to the gym the next day? It happens with me all the time, and I am pretty committed to my workouts. What do we do then?

Well, if I had been Keith's trainer, I would have asked him to rest. Did you know sleep loss increases the risk of injuries by decreasing balance and postural control? A bad night's sleep can lead to deteriorated functioning, difficulty concentrating, and slower reaction time[37,38].

Yes, most Americans are sleep deprived, getting less than six hours a night on average[39]. I would rather sleep more.

In today's world, people have started taking the famous saying "**no pain, no gain**" quite literally. They consider it cool to go to sleep at midnight and be there for their gruesome CrossFit session at 5:00 am. Not my style. I instead replace the saying with "*no brain*, **no gain**" and listen to my body more. The choice is yours!

The bottom line is that performing a spilt, which requires you to be in the gym five to six times a week, becomes impractical for most of us. However, with FBX routines you are working out no more than three days a week, so obstacles like the ones Keith faced in our example are literally reduced or nonexistent. You can simply skip the days you are not up for a workout and compensate with a quick HIIT session (or even go for a long walk) and postpone your weights session until the next day. I don't want something so regimented that it needs to be done in a particular way. I want a training schedule with more flexibility to suit my motivation and energy levels, and of course, my lifestyle. In Neghar Fonooni's words, "**Hustle one day, and flow the other.**" That's how I'd like to function.

Yes, there are individuals I know who are in the gym every day no matter what comes up, and I applaud their commitment and dedication. But there are definitely times these people ignore the signal their body is giving them, which may lead to overtraining. Over time, overtraining can be detrimental with a nasty injury waiting to happen. Working out is a stress to the body. I would rather be conservative with exercise protocols than overdo it.

3. FBX workouts are sustainable.

When I shared my three-times-a-week routine with my friends and clients in the gym, of course they were reluctant first, but once they were following the routine for a while, they really started to enjoy it. They'd mention how they really look forward to their workouts. Whenever they came to the gym they were full of energy and gave their best, their poundage started to increase and results were there to show.

When you know that you only have to be in the gym three times a week, you are more likely to be consistent with your workouts. Working out will become a lifestyle, not a compulsion, and you will be less likely to give up. Over time, this will mean better results. And your wife will be thankful too!

4. FBX workouts creates a real, natural-looking body.

Fabulous bodies are not chiseled to perfection. The FBX routine won't get you first place in a physique competition, but then, the majority of us simply want to look good in a shirt, so why do we want more isolated training to hit our muscle from every angle? Here, the idea is to look good and **optimize our gene expression** in as little time as possible. FBX workouts eliminate most isolated exercises, which I deem to be useless. The focus is on compound functional movements that mimic our real, lifelike movement in order to grow stronger in those. If you do this, you will never go wrong, and I promise you will build a physique that will turn heads in the shortest time possible.

One other benefit with FBX is that you are not likely to skip a body part—the result is a more balanced looking physique. With spilt routine workouts, I have witnessed people conveniently skipping body parts they are not fond of (calves, neck, thighs, back, shoulders, in this order). In most cases, *mirror muscles* (chest and arms) are worked the most, which creates a rather imbalanced physique.

5. **FBX workouts save you money**.

Naturally with fewer workout days, you will be less inclined to have post-workout shakes; instead you will consume your daily quota of protein mainly from whole foods. My whey protein consumption usually drops on the day I don't workout, though this is not always the case—it depends upon my meal plan for that day. But overall my supplement consumption has definitely been reduced since I started doing FBX workouts.

6. **FBX workouts save you time**.

My total workout time (including HIIT and yoga) is no more than three to six hours a week. Many spilt routine advocates also vouch for the same number of hours. Well, I disagree!

With every workout, we want to give our best and possibly progress, right? It could be progression with a little more weight on your squat, or it could be decreasing the rest intervals between your sets. Whatever the case, progressing requires lot of mental strength and planning ahead—pre-workout meals, getting a good night's sleep the night before, etc. I sometimes take a power nap right before my workout, which definitely helps me.

All this takes time, as does getting ready to go to the gym and time in traffic to get there and back. It can take a good three hours or so overall to complete a one-hour workout.

For anyone working out five or six times weekly, this would mean anywhere from 15 – 18 hours per week.

With FBX workouts, my clients have reported a total time commitment of no more than 10 hours including their traveling time. That's a total time commitment of just 6 percent of the total number of hours in a week!

Note: If you love going to the gym five or six times a week, that's awesome! If you feel that you can easily devote 15 – 18 per week to workouts, and going to gym is something you look forward to, that's great; by all means go ahead. I won't stop you. **But please consider my point here:** I don't support working out with weights six times per week. Equal importance needs to be given to HIIT and to yoga or other balance protocols, including a comprehensive flexibility regime. All you gym lovers can perform these other movements at your health club instead of your home.

We all want to optimize the effort versus benefit ratio, right? We all want exceptional results in the least time possible. It's possible to get exceptional results working out only three times a week. You will never need to do more!

If you have spent a lot of time on split trainings and more workout days rather than fewer, you may feel attached to your routine despite much frustration. Have the courage to know that whatever hasn't gotten you results in the past will never get you results in the future. Break away from the norm, and stop following what others are doing; it will get you nothing except misery and failure.

Honestly ask yourself: Is there any more time to waste?

Start new, with more passion and with a state of faith. Apply what you have read in this book diligently with proper planning and persistence, and victory will be yours. Then you will be a believer.

CHAPTER 10:
SELECTION OF MOVEMENTS: FOLLOWING THE 80/20 RULE

Before we get to the workouts themselves, let's first discuss selection of movements. Staying true to our first law (less is more, the 80/20 Pareto principle), 20 percent of exercises in the gym will provide us with 80 percent of the results. This 20 percent consists of the following primary movements, which pretty much covers your entire body:

1. Parallel-grip deadlift
2. Barbell squat
3. Military press (seated or standing)
4. Front lat pulldown
5. Weighted pullup
6. Incline barbell bench press
7. Weighted dip

Remember, these are the exercises/movements that will give you more than 80 percent of your results. Learn them, re-establish the feel, set strength targets, and you'll see yourself transform in the shortest time possible.

However, just like supplements assist our wholesome diet in keeping us healthy, there are 15 – 20 supplementary exercises that will help you develop a proportionate, symmetrical and fabulous body, but we will use these supplementary exercises sparingly.

Now let's briefly discuss each body part and the exercises that will come together to form a workout routine for that part.

Thighs

The two mass builders that will work your thighs better than any exercise out there are **squats** and **parallel-grip deadlifts**. Initially, they may seem tough and intimidating, but once you start doing them, you will love them, and when you start getting stronger doing them, you will love them even more.

You will become so passionate about doing squats and p.g deadlifts that people around you will start doing them too. Yes, they are addictive, as they have decades of history of building ultimate male physiques behind them. However there are barriers, myths, and common concerns that come up for a weight lifter when these exercises are discussed.

1. **I have a weak lower back and I may hurt myself if I perform squats/p.g deadlifts**. The beauty about progressive weight training is that it is for the weak and for the strong. Squats and p.g. deadlifts actually make your lower back strong—very strong. If you have a weak lower back, you have even more reason to include squats and p.g deadlifts in your workouts!

2. **Squats and p.g deadlifts are too tough for me**. Honestly, if you think you cannot bear the discomfort of heavy weights and compound exercises like these, please choose moderate activities like yoga, swimming, or any sport—they are good enough to keep you in shape. But if you want to build a lean, admirable physique that people stop to admire, you

need to pay the price, and that price comes in the form of some discomfort.

3. **I am not flexible enough to perform these movements.** Performing squats and p.g deadlifts will make you flexible. Weight training in general makes you flexible; if you exercise with good technique and with complete range of motion you will become as flexible as you need to be[40].

4. **I can get good results without doing squats and p.g deadlifts**. Squats and p.g deadlifts are the core movements of any strength training program, and if any program excludes these exercises, it is missing tons and tons of benefits. Squats and p.g deadlifts are like the engine of my program; without them, the FBX training system will not be complete.

Note: In a few cases where individuals have slipped discs and other clinical lower back issues, there are alternatives to these exercises that I recommend. However, if you simply suffer from lower back pain, its main cause is likely chronic sitting; this should not be used as an excuse not to do these exercises.

I have written long articles backed by scientific studies done on these exercises. You can read them on my blog fabulousbody.com:

The Ultimate Guide to Squatting

The Ultimate Guide to Parallel Grip Deadlifting (Be particularly sure to read this article, as parallel grip deadlifts are a great functional exercise and could be a good solution for individuals with long limbs for whom squatting with good range of motion is an issue.)

Read and study the articles, then apply them, starting light and building up the correct technique, and I promise you squats and p.g deadlifts will become your best friends in the gym.

Exercises for Thighs

Barbell squat
Parallel grip deadlift

For anyone who is suffering from clinical lower back problems:

Leg press
Dumbbell lunge

Note: We generally believe, that barbell squats and parallel grip deadlifts are meant to train your thighs. I disagree! Yes, it's true that both squats and parallel grip deadlifts directly target your leg muscles, but they also train your lower back and core muscles. Since leg muscles are the largest in the body, there is a huge hormonal burst after doing these exercises that helps in gaining tremendous amounts of muscles in the fastest time possible.

Shoulders

For shoulders, the military press is the name of the game. It's the ultimate mass builder for shoulders. However, you can do many variations. You can do them standing or seated (to give your lower back a break from all the squats and p.g deadlifts), and instead of a barbell you can use dumbbells. What about lateral raise and posterior raise? Well, these are not mass builders and should not be your priority especially when you are a beginner/intermediate or trying to build mass.

Exercises for Shoulders

Seated Military Press
Seated dumbbell press
Dumbbell lateral raise
Dumbbell posterior raise

Chest

Honestly, I am not a big fan of building too much chest muscle. Overbuilt pectorals makes you look more like a bodybuilder, plus it overshadows the development of your shoulders and makes them look smaller.

Also note that chest muscles only form part of your chest circumference (CC). The size of your rib box and your latissimus dorsi are part of CC. In chapter 5, we discussed the golden ratio. My target has always been a CC at least 1.4 times my waist, which gives it the perfect V shape. That's a difference of at least 11 inches! The best exercises to build your chest are incline dumbbell press and/or weighted dips. Dumbbell flyers are to chest what lateral raises are to the shoulders, so focus on your primary exercises first.

Exercises for Chest

Incline Barbell Bench press
Incline Dumbbell Press
Weighed Chest Dip
Flat Dumbbell Bench Press
Flat Barbell Bench Press

Upper Back

Pull-ups are by far the best compound exercise for your upper back. If you are strong enough to pull your body weight at least 10 times, buy a weighed belt and increase resistance as you go along. However, if you are still not that strong (don't worry, the majority of men in the gym can't even lift their bodyweight a few times), you can start with lat pulldowns until you get strong enough to start doing pull-ups.

Exercises for Back

Weighed Pull-up
Weighed Chin-up
Front lat pulldown
Single arm dumbbell row
Seated Cable Row

Arm

The majority of average Joes going to the gym will easily devote a day per week to working out their arms, especially their biceps. They will perform preacher curls, kickbacks, concentrates, and all sorts of fancy but useless exercises to pump their arm muscles. You look at them after six months, and their arm size is still the same (some of them may even have lost some size). What they are unaware of is that when they perform shoulder and chest exercises, their triceps get a good workout. When they work their back, their biceps get worked out. Personally, I have hardly worked out my arms in over a year now, and I think I have gained an inch or so. How? By increasing my lean weight of course.

To increase one inch on your arms you need to increase your muscular weight by 10 pounds, and the way to do that is to perform compound exercises. Still, I have included a few exercises for your arms in FBX workouts.

Exercises for Arms

Incline dumbbell curl
Barbell curl

Seated Dumbbell Curl
Triceps pushdown
Close-Grip Barbell Bench Press
Seated Triceps Press

Calves

Beautifully developed calves give the whole body (especially your lower half) a complete look. Still, they are the most neglected body part, and they can easily be covered by not wearing shorts, so the vanity muscles (chest and arms) get the most attention.

Calves are usually an afterthought, and one usually perform one or two sets of halfhearted sets of calf exercise. Lucky ones with good genetics don't really feel the need to work out the calves. Over time, I have made my calves a priority, and I give them more attention than my arms! I am obsessed about building a balanced and pleasing physique; it's one of the main goals of Fabulous Body. Calves are utterly stubborn muscles, and you need to include a lot of specialization work if you really want to build them up.

Exercises for Calves

Standing calf raise
Seated calves raise
Donkey calf raise

Neck

Again, genetics play a very important role. I have friends who have never done any weight training or any direct neck work, yet they have big necks. When you wear a suit, your neck is visible, and if you have a pencil neck, no matter how much muscles you have beneath that suit, you are going to look awkward. As an ectomorph, I have always had an underdeveloped neck, and I do a lot of isolation work to bring it in balance with my arms and calves.

Steve Reeves had the most pleasing physique ever. His measurements of neck, arms and calves were all 18 inches! Again, it's a personal preference, but I can promise you one thing: If you bring your neck, arms and calves measurement in line, you will dramatically enhance the "pleasing" aspect of your physique. A thick strong neck also signals physical strength and vigor, and it can save you from potential injury. Ask any boxer or rugby player about the importance of a strong neck.

Exercises for Neck

Neck Flexion
Neck Extension

Note: You can use your hand as a form of resistance, however I would suggest a neck harness (Harbinger has good products) to really build a massive neck.

Abdominals

FBX workouts are built on compound exercises using dumbbells and barbells, which stimulates your abdominals to a T. Still I have included some direct work to strengthen and build them further.

Exercises for Abs

Basic crunch
Oblique crunch
Leg raise
Knee/Hip Raise on Parallel Bar

Lower Back

Your lower back will get enough work from squats, deadlifts, and military press (if you perform them standing), still I would recommend performing stiff leg deadlift once every two weeks to give your lower back a really good dose of training.

Exercises for Lower Back

Stiff leg deadlift
Hyperextension
Cobra pose

CHAPTER 11:
INTENSITY: THE BIG-DADDY OF PRINCIPLES

At the end of every workout, I rate my intensity on a scale of 1 – 10. Between 6 and 8 means that I pushed myself only just so far. After the workout, I would feel that I could have done more.

Anything above 8 is pretty intensive. It means that I gave my all in the workout. After the workout, I feel tired but also rejuvenated! With above 8 intensity, I know that my metabolism will be at an all-time high for few days because of growth stimulation in my muscles. At this intensity, I am content.

The scale method is a decent way to judge your intensity levels. But if you're serious about your training, you should go a step further (by keeping a training diary), imagine Michael Phelps' coaches relying on a scale of 1 – 10 instead of a stopwatch. God bless them!

Intensity is defined as the "effort" you put in your workouts. One of the best ways to increase intensity is to increase poundage, ideally at every workout. Say I deadlifted 300 pounds on Monday, and in my next workout on Friday I added 3 pounds. Provided that all the variables remain the same (reps, sets, the sequence of the exercises, and the rest intervals), I have increased my intensity.

Other methods to increase intensity include increasing the number of reps, sets, or even the total volume of your workouts. The variables you tweak to change your intensity also depend on what you are training for, i.e. to increase in muscular mass, to lose fat, or simply for cardio fitness.

Does this mean that you should work hard and give your all every time at the gym?

NO! Although training hard is essential to building a fabulous body, you should not train intensely at every workout every week throughout the year.

The correct application of effort is the essence of intensity variation.

You should take it easy when starting a new routine or at the start of a new cycle of a familiar routine. Also, beginners should not be concerned with intensity variations for at least six months. Further, I have not met anyone who can train with serious weights throughout the year. That's why I have built modifications into the FBX Gain and Cut workout routines.

There are six main variables by which one can vary their intensity levels (although the amount of weight used is the most important one). Let's discuss each variable briefly and figure out how they can be combined together to form a workout routine that is personalized and customizable according to one's goals.

The six variables are:

1. Number of reps
2. Amount of weight used
3. Tempo of each rep
4. Number of sets
5. Rest interval between sets

6. Total volume/muscle group/week

Amount of Weight and Number of Repetitions

To understand the relationship between the amount of weight and number of repetitions, consider the concept of 1 rep max—the maximum weight one can lift in a given movement. To test it, we use sub maximal options (which you can do
here: www.exrx.net/Calculators/OneRepMax.html)

The following table shows the relationship between number of reps and the amount of weight lifted[41]:

REPS (Estimated Reps at Percent of 1 Repetition Maximum)	Brzycki % 1RM	Baechle % 1RM	dos Remedios % 1RM
1	100	100	100
2	95	95	92
3	90	93	90
4	88	90	87
5	86	87	85
6	83	85	82
7	80	83	
8	78	80	75
9	76	77	
10	75	75	70
11	72		

REPS (Estimated Reps at Percent of 1 Repetition Maximum)	Brzycki % 1RM	Baechle % 1RM	dos Remedios % 1RM
12	70	67	65
15		65	60

A repetition is a complete movement through a particular exercise.

Repetitions can be classified into three basic ranges:

Rep Category	Rep Range	Energy System Used
LOW	1 – 4	Phosphocreatine System
MODERATE	5 – 12	Anaerobic Glycolysis
HIGH	12+	Anaerobic Glycolysis/Oxidative System

To **build muscles you need to lift weights** between 70 – 85 percent of your 1 rep max, which creates greatest hypertrophy. If you notice in the table above, **this means you would do 5 – 12 repetitions for every set.**

A meta-analysis[42] of 140 studies was done in 2003 in relation to strength training, and the researchers concluded that *"training with a mean intensity of 60 percent (15 reps) of one repetition maximum elicits maximal gains in untrained individuals, whereas 80 percent (6 – 7 reps) is most effective in those who are trained."*

Now, some fitness experts swear by the low rep range (3 – 5), whereas others advocate a more moderate range (7 – 12). Which is the best for optimal hypertrophy (a fancy term for muscle growth)? To answer this question, we need to figure out what exactly muscle hypertrophy is and what types exist.

Muscle hypertrophy is increase in the size of skeletal muscles. Hypertrophy is of two types: **Myofibrillar hypertrophy** is increase in the size and number of the myofibril contractile proteins actin and myosin. When they grow in number within a muscle fiber, the amount of force that can be produced goes up too. Heavy lifting (80-100% of 1 rep max) induces this type of hypertrophy. Focusing on this kind of hypertrophy gives you rock hard, dense muscles.

On the other hand, **sarcoplasmic hypertrophy** is increase in non-contractile components (collagen, glycogen, water, etc.) in the muscle cell. This type of hypertrophy may result in greater muscle bulk without increases in strength. Moderate weights (70 – 80 percent of 1 rep max) induces this type of hypertrophy. Focusing on this kind of hypertrophy gives you those puffy bodybuilder muscles.

Recall muscle building principle #1, where we established that creating muscular tension is more important than creating metabolic stress when it comes to triggering muscle growth. We know that to create muscular tension we need to lift heavy weights with a low to moderate rep range (3 – 7). Similarly, to create more metabolic stress we need to lift weights with a moderate rep range (8 – 12). So what's the **optimal rep range** for muscle growth?

The optimal rep range for muscle growth is 5 – 7 reps.

Our main focus will be to get as strong as possible with this rep range (which is good enough for some sarcoplasmic hypertrophy as well).

Now, in my experience, working out with a rep range of 5 – 7 throughout the year is close to impossible for most trainees and can be very mentally challenging (especially for beginners and intermediates), and that's the reason some kind of periodization is essential.

The variety of a higher rep scheme (8 – 10 reps) will add an element of enjoyment and fun and can be a nice break from all that heavy lifting.

The bottom line is **lifting moderate weight is fun, whereas lifting heavier weight is tough**. Most trainees focus on the former and end up with a mediocre physique. Over the long term, your muscle growth will depend on how strong you have gotten.

If you can bench press with 250 pounds, perform a pull-up (with a 75 – 100 pound weighted belt) and squat 300 pounds for a few reps, you can't help but have a spectacular physique.

Note: The majority of people don't maintain a training diary because they think it's hard work to do so, or they simply think it's not important. The above science-based discussion will be futile if you don't know whether the weights you are lifting for the required rep range is too light or too heavy for you.

If the weight is too light and you don't maintain a training diary, chances are high that you will select a weight that is too light for you when you want to perform 5 – 7 reps. Once you are into the set, you realize that you can easily perform 12 reps with that weight. What do you do? Of course, you increase the weight, which enables you to perform somewhere close to 6 reps. You give your all with this X amount and you perform 8 reps (you take this set to failure) and you are happy. What are the chances that you come back next week and remember your 8 RM weight if you have not logged it? You start to guess. Over time, what really happens is you are performing far too many sets where you are not achieving progressive overload, which then short changes your results.

Bottom line: Always maintain a training diary.

Tempo of a Rep

When I played golf for the first time a few years back, I became really good at it, although I didn't continued for very long. But in that short stint of few months, my approach shots always landed on the greens. In fact, a few members of the club even complimented me, suggesting that had I started early, I could have played professionally. (I was on cloud nine.) My coach videotaped me the first time I took a swing and said that I am a natural athlete, and that hitting over 300 yards with a driver wouldn't be an issue for me. But he clearly stated (keeping his eyes on my bulging biceps when saying this) that it's not brutal strength that will get the ball to reach its destination but rather the technique. He said I needed to establish the "feel" of the sweet spot when hitting the ball.

A sweet spot is present in every sport from cricket to tennis, and lifting weights is no exception.

In my experience working in the gym environment, I can honestly say that the majority of trainees use faulty technique when doing any exercise. They load too much weight, they use momentum to complete their reps, and they compensate by bringing other muscles into play. For example, a common error when performing a lat pulldown is elevating the shoulders, which reduces the effect on lats. There are certain checkpoints when performing any exercises, and I would strongly recommend that you master them before loading up the bar. I have provided links to external third party sites, which will assist you in performing every exercise effectively and safely.

Ideally, the concentric phase should be 1 – 2 seconds, whereas the eccentric phase should be around 2 – 3 seconds, although my suggestion is to not focus on timings too much and simply go with controlled reps. A controlled rep is lifting weights without using momentum, which also establishes superior communication between your brain and muscles. This can only happen when you concentrate on the muscles being worked and not too much on how much weight you are lifting.

Ideally one should enter into a meditative state and shut everything out. It becomes difficult to do so if you are working out in a crowded gym. I have listed four suggestions in chapter 15 that will dramatically increase your concentration levels and focus while working out in a gym.

How many sets per exercise?

A set is a group of repetitions. Two sets of maximum effort are far more effective than one, and it appears that three sets are slightly more beneficial than two.

Here is a quote from the most admired bodybuilder of the twentieth century, Steve Reeves: "If you cannot stimulate your muscles in three sets for an exercise, you are doing it wrong."

Add warmup sets if the particular exercise is early in your workout or you are working out a different muscle group and you are set. You will not need to do more. One of the most common mistakes people make in the gym is they perform far too may sets before they actually come to their main sets (where progressive overload happens).

For example, say a lifter can squat 250 pounds for 10 reps, and this time he wants to beat this number and squat 255 pounds for 10 reps. This is how a typical trainee goes about this (note that the squats are performed after he has already done a shoulder session):

1. He performs a warmup set of 120 pounds for 15 reps.
2. He then does a second warmup set of 180 pounds for 10 reps.
3. And one more set of 200 pounds for 8 reps.
4. Then he adds a set of 225 pounds and performs 6 reps.
5. And finally he comes to his 255 pounds and is not able to do more than 6 reps!

Can you spot the mistake?

He has already used up lot of his energy by performing a shoulder session, and then he performs four sets with high reps before his overload set, which fatigues his muscles further. By the time to give his best shot, he is already very tired.

What would I have done?

I would also perform four warmup sets of 20 percent of my target weight (50 pounds for 10 – 12 reps), 40 percent (100 pounds for 8 – 10 reps), 70 percent (175 pounds for 5 – 6 reps), and 90 percent (230 pounds for 1 – 2 reps). Notice I am gradually increasing my weights so that my muscles, ligaments, and tendons get used to the weights, and **I am decreasing the reps,** I am doing so that I don't fatigue my muscles. Then I am good to go all out for three sets of progressive overload.

Now, the question is should you do this for every exercise? NO! You should do it for the first exercise in the muscle group and when you change the muscle group. For example, if you are training shoulders and legs on one day, then perform the warmup routine for military press, but not for the lateral raises that comes after the press. Similarly, if you are performing chest exercises and then move to back exercises, perform the warmup for the first back exercise only.

In the FBX system of training, you are trying to beat your overload set from the last workout in **all three sets**. I can assure you that you will never ever feel undertrained; in fact, in most cases you may even have to lower the entire volume of your workouts as the intensity will be high.

Putting your mind on the muscle (not on the weight being lifted) and establishing a controlled movement during the entire range of motion is imperative. If the quality of every rep in the set is perfect, you won't need more than three sets per exercise ever.

Rest Intervals in Between Sets

A rest interval is the time you take between each set to recuperate. Rest between sets should be at least one minute and no more than five minutes. No difference in terms of growth and strength increase has been shown between taking a one-minute or five-minute rest; the choice is yours. Some may argue that shorter rest intervals (less than one minute) generate significant metabolic stress, which heightens anabolic processes like release of HGH. This is true, but a minute or less doesn't give sufficient time for the lifter to regain muscular strength, which then impairs his ability to lift the required poundage. Therefore the greater muscular stress is offset by a subsequent decrease in the amount of weight lifted, i.e. there is less muscular tension.

If you are lifting weights near 80 – 85 percent of your 1 rep max (5 – 7 reps), you need to take at least a two to four minute break, which results in full recovery of ATP/CP. However, if you are in the fat loss stage, you will still lift heavy weights with 8 – 10 reps and focus on taking only one to two minute rests, which results in 75 – 80 percent ATP/CP recovery. This kind of training is similar to circuit training and can be a good variation to your workout. That's why I advocate a low to moderate rep range for the FBX-Gain workouts and a moderate rep range for the FBX-Cut workouts.

Total volume per muscle group/week

Volume can be defined as the total amount of work within a specified period of time. Total volume goes down as the intensity of your workouts increases. With heavy weights you need more time to recover between workouts. Unlike many spilt routines, where volumes are massive, **I prescribe a low volume model with high intensity compound exercises.** Naturally with high intensity more recovery is needed, which is why you will only be working out three times a week.

Approximate Training volume for most bodybuilding programs:

TRAINING EXPERIENCE	TOTAL SETS FOR MAJOR MUSCLE GROUP PER WEEK	TOTAL SETS FOR MINOR MUSCLE GROUP PER WEEK
INTERMEDIATE	18—24	12
ADVANCED	24—32	18

Training volume for FBX workouts:

TRAINING EXPERIENCE	TOTAL SETS FOR MAJOR MUSCLE GROUP PER WEEK	TOTAL SETS FOR MINOR MUSCLE GROUP PER WEEK
INTERMEDIATE	7—9	4
ADVANCED	9—12	6

WORKOUT ROUTINES

All the FBX workouts are listed in the bonus report which can be downloaded at the end of this book.

CHAPTER 12: SUPPLEMENTING WITH HIIT

High Intensity Interval Training (HIIT) is a form of cardiovascular training performed on any cardio machine like a treadmill or cross trainer. It can also be done using calisthenics (like Tabata) or even via a swim. HIIT alternates periods of short intense anaerobic exercise with less intense recovery periods. Sessions usually vary in length from 4 – 20 minutes.

How to perform HIIT

ACSM Guidelines on HIIT are as follows[43]:

When developing a HIIT program, we need to consider the duration, intensity, and frequency of the work intervals and the length of recovery intervals.

First we need to calculate maximum heart rate (MHR): Maximum heart rate can be calculated by subtracting your age from 220. So if you are 30 years old, your MHR is 220 - 30 = 190.

During the high intensity work interval, your heart rate should be 80 percent or greater of your estimated maximum heart rate. A good indicator of your intensity is a talk test. If you are unable to carry on a conversation with someone, you are exercising "very hard" and you can carry on until you are not able to go further for even a few seconds. This will vary according to your fitness level.

The intensity of the recovery interval should be 40 – 50 percent of your maximum heart rate. This would be an activity level you would be very comfortable with and during which you could carry on a conversation with relative ease. For more accurate estimates, consider buying a heart rate monitor or a Fitbit band.

The relationship between the work and recovery intervals is very important when designing a HIIT session. Many studies use a specific ratio of exercise to recovery to improve the different energy systems of the body. For example, a ratio of 1:1 might be a 3-minute hard work (or high intensity) bout followed by a 3-minute recovery (or low intensity) bout. These 1:1 interval workouts are often 3, 4, or 5 minutes followed by an equal time in recovery.

Another popular HIIT training protocol is called the "spring interval training method." With this type of program the exerciser does about 30 seconds of "sprint or near full out effort" followed by 4 to 4.5 minutes of recovery. This combination of exercises can be repeated three to five times. These higher intensity work efforts are typically shorter bouts (30 seconds with sprint interval training).

How many times a week can you do a HIIT workout?

HIIT workouts are exhaustive and require a longer recovery period than regular cardio workouts.

With FBX we will be focusing on heavy weightlifting two to three times a week; therefore more than three HIIT sessions of 20 minutes each can become a challenge. Well, it all depends upon one's recuperative power (which in turn depends on genetics, sleep, nutrition etc.). Still, in my experience more than three sessions of HIIT per week for a serious weightlifter is pushing the limit.

I encourage you to perform HIIT not in the gym, but outdoors. There are two main reasons for this. First, working out in the open provides exposure to sunlight, which stimulates Vitamin D synthesis in the epidermis. Recall that Fabulous Body Law #6 talks about the importance of Vitamin D and why deficiency of this vitamin is a common strong risk factor for many health concerns, including cardiovascular disease. Second, it has been demonstrated that outdoor exercise decreases emotional stress and improves mood to a greater extent than indoor exercise[44].

Adding a swim session two times a week has been the best decision I have made regarding my health in the past year or so (my pool is out in the open). I enjoy and prefer swimming over performing HIIT on any cardio machine, which I find to be somewhat boring.

Exceptional Benefits of High Intensity Interval Training over Regular Cardio

HIIT has been shown to significantly increase both aerobic and anaerobic fitness. HIIT also significantly lowers insulin resistance and results in a number of skeletal adaptations that enhance skeletal muscle fat oxidation and improved glucose tolerance[45].

HIIT boosts massive production of HGH and testosterone, which helps build muscles and improve tone. Did you know that performing high intensity training activates the super-fast fibers (white muscle fibers), which are key to producing growth hormone (the anti-aging hormone)

A study also indicates that it's possible to achieve a fiber type transformation with high intensity training[46].

Another 12-week controlled study[47] in Denmark of high-intensity interval walking for patients with type 2 diabetes showed that it was better at helping to control blood glucose levels than continuous moderate exercise, even though the same number of calories was expended by both groups. Interval training also was more effective at enhancing physical fitness and reducing body fat relative to lean muscle tissue.

Note: HIIT protocols are extremely challenging and may not be for everyone. One has to be highly motivated to tolerate the accompanying discomfort.

In a recent report[48] in the American College of Sports Medicine's Health & Fitness Journal, Dr. Little; his wife, Mary E. Jung, also at the University of British Columbia; and Marcus W. Kilpatrick of the University of South Florida wrote that HIIT "is only appropriate for low-risk individuals, moderate-risk individuals who have been cleared for vigorous intensities by a medical professional, and high-risk individuals who are under direct medical supervision during exercise training."

Any movement is better than none. Yes, there are overwhelming numbers of recent studies showing that HIIT protocols are not limited to athletes anymore. Further, HIIT can yield a broad range of physiological gains, **often in less time** than steady state cardio. I am not against steady-state cardio per se but I want to alert people who rely on it completely and are doing it excessively that it can cause muscular imbalances and loss of muscle mass.

For me, performing high intensity training like heavy weightlifting and HIIT can take a toll on my mental strength too. Sometimes, taking it easy on a cardio machine while watching TV is a much welcome break and can actually be rejuvenating. But only sometimes!

CHAPTER 13:
SURPRISING BENEFITS OF INCORPORATING 10,000 STEPS IN YOUR DAILY LIFESTYLE

Is there more to do when it comes to staying fit?

YES! There are dozens of studies which clearly states that besides high intensity workouts, one needs an overall active lifestyle to be healthy.

According to this meta-analysis of eighteen studies which included 794,577 participants, being sedentary (usually classified as taking fewer than 3000 steps per day) was associated with a 112 percent increased risk of diabetes and 147 percent increased risk of cardiovascular disease[49].

According to Tom Rath, the bestselling author of *Eat, Move, Sleep*, which had sold more than 6 million copies:

"Sitting more than six hours a day greatly increases your risk of an early death. No matter how much you exercise, eat well, avoid smoking, or add other healthy habits, excessive sitting will cause problems." Rath further states that as soon as you sit down, electrical activity in your leg muscles shuts off. The number of calories you burn drops to one per minute, and enzyme production, which helps break down fat, drops by 90 percent. After two hours of sitting, your good cholesterol drops by 20 percent. Perhaps this explains why people with desk jobs have twice the rate of cardiovascular disease."

Another study, this one conducted by Rory Heath and published in the *British Medical Journal* states[50]:

1. *During waking hours, 65 percent of an average person's day is spent sedentary; that is 9 – 10 hours for adults*

2. *Sitting at work accounts for 60 percent of total daily sitting on a weekday, but even on weekends people still sit for 8 hours*

3. *Positive associations between cancer risk and sedentary behavior exist:*
   - Lung cancer risk increases by 54 percent.
   - Uterine cancer risk increases by 66 percent.
   - Colon cancer risk increases by 30 percent.

I took this information seriously and incorporated it in my FBX Training System.

The concept of 10,000 steps a day is brilliant, and I feel everyone should be consciously focused on reaching this target daily. The first question that came to my mind is whether 10,000 steps is enough, so I googled it, and this is the first thing that came up:

*The average person's stride length is approximately 2.5 feet long. That means it takes just over 2,000 steps to walk one mile, and **10,000 steps is close to 5 miles**. A sedentary person may only average 1,000 – 3,000 steps a day*[51].

Then again, is 5 miles enough?

Recall James H. O'Keefe's comprehensive research on the activity of hunter-gatherers. He writes:

"A large amount of daily, light-to-moderate activity such as walking was required. Although the distances covered would have varied widely according to hunting and foraging

routines, cultures, weather, seasons, ages, etc., most estimates indicate that the average daily distances covered were in the range of 6 – 16 km."

The equivalent of 6 – 16 km is approximately 3 – 10 miles. What we need to do is focus on taking at least 5,000 steps every day and gradually increase it to 10,000 steps.

Here are few things you can start doing every day to come close to taking 10,000 steps:

First, know how many steps you take. There are many apps that you can download on your smart phone to track your steps, however since you won't be carrying your phone everywhere, these apps will underestimate the number of steps you take. Another cheap option is a pedometer. If you want to spend a bit extra, buy a fitness tracking device like Fitbit which not only tracks your steps but also suggests the quantity and quality of your sleep.

Be sure you are taking at least 5,000 steps daily. If you are taking fewer, you are sedentary. Better yet, aim for a minimum of 7,000 steps or more. By making the following changes, you can average between 7,000 and 10,000:

1. Make walking part of your daily routine. Now, for most of us, sitting in front of the computer is totally unavoidable. Since the day I realized sitting can be that harmful, **I never sit for more than 15 minutes at a time**. I often stand when I work. (I recently got a custom-made standing desk, and I feel it's one of the best health investments I have made so far.) Most of my work is creative as it entails writing content, and walking in between work sessions really helps me. Ideas flow more freely, and I absolutely love the way this whole thing works out. I have easily added close to 3,000 steps more than my previous average of

3,000 plus at least a few hours of standing (and we all know standing burns more calories than sitting).

2. Find ways to add steps to your daily routine. My two-year-old has tremendously contributed to adding close to 2,000 steps, as he often enters my home office. He demands lot of attention as every child does, and I am more than happy to take frequent breaks to play with him. (If you don't have an infant at home, get a dog.)

3. Make small changes in your routine. Whenever I watch TV, I make it a point to get up when a commercial comes on. I often take the stairs (I live on the 8th floor), and whenever I get a phone call, I stand while I talk. Cooking and things like that add more time standing. In fact, since I purchased my Fitbit device, I am hell-bent on reaching my daily target of 10,000 steps, and I think it's gradually becoming a solid lifestyle habit.

What if you don't have the luxury of standing up and moving around while at the office?

In this case, drink more water so you will need to take more frequent trips to the bathroom! (Just kidding.)

If you have absolutely no other option, a new position while sitting is always better than the old position, so keep fidgeting. To maintain a neutral spine, buy a laptop stand and raise the level of your laptop (this has the added benefit of keeping your machine from heating up too much). You can also do certain stretches. The whole idea is to keep moving even when you are sitting.

Take home message: The human body was designed to move. Sitting puts you in an unnatural position, putting stress on your entire kinetic chain, which leads to muscular imbalances like tight hip flexors, rounded shoulders, and a forward neck. This can also cause breathing problems and put severe stress on your lower back. Everyone reading this should know that chronic sitting is a real threat that should be taken seriously.

CHAPTER 14:
FLEXIBILITY AND NEUROMOTOR PROTOCOL

And now, we have come to the last leg of the FBX training system without which this system would not be complete.

In this section, I will throw some fancy terms at you. The majority of readers will be unaware of these terms, and that's OK! Just like you don't need to understand how electricity is created to enjoy its benefits, you don't need to know these terms; you simply need to include these protocols in your workouts to gain full benefits. So brace yourself and let's get started.

Again, recall James O'Keefe's research on hunter-gatherers, which states:

Their routines promoted aerobic endurance, flexibility, and strength, thereby providing them with multifaceted fitness. This varied pattern of movement would have also conferred resiliency and reduced the likelihood of injury, allowing them to hunt and forage without major interruptions.

Also recall the ACSM guidelines:

Flexibility Exercise

☐ *Adults should do flexibility exercises at least two or three days each week to improve range of motion.*

☐ *Each stretch should be held for 10 – 30 seconds to the point of tightness or slight discomfort.*

- ☐ *Repeat each stretch two to four times, accumulating 60 seconds per stretch.*

- ☐ *Static, dynamic, ballistic, and PNF stretches are all effective.*

- ☐ *Flexibility exercise is most effective when the muscle is warm. Try light aerobic activity or a hot bath to warm the muscles before stretching.*

Neuromotor Exercise

- ☐ *Neuromotor exercise (sometimes called "functional fitness training") is recommended for two or three days per week.*

- ☐ *Exercises should involve motor skills (balance, agility, coordination, and gait), proprioceptive exercise training, and multifaceted activities (tai ji and yoga) to improve physical function and prevent falls in older adults.*

- ☐ *20 – 30 minutes per day is appropriate for neuromotor exercise.*

We need a total of **1 – 1.5 hours per week of flexibility and neuromotor exercises spread over two or three sessions**.

Besides looking good and being healthy, being *functional* is essential. What do I mean by ***functional***? Being functional in practical terms means that you are completely free of any pains or aches and can perform everyday movements like tying your shoelaces, getting out of a car, playing a sport, and performing a parallel squat with relative ease.

Unfortunately, with today's modern lifestyle, most people are de-conditioned—A state of lost physical fitness, which may include muscle imbalances, decreased flexibility and/or a lack of core and joint stability, and one of the main reasons for this is chronic sitting, as we discussed in the previous section. Chronic sitting results in common muscle imbalances: forward head, protracted shoulders, anterior pelvic tilt, etc.

Most people treat fitness as an event and not a lifestyle. After a prolonged period of living a sedentary lifestyle (where they get de-conditioned), they get excited one day and decide to lose 20 pounds in a month. They either start playing a sport or start a routine of chronic cardio and weight training. What they don't understand is that this creates major stress on their joints, which might lead to a nasty injury that is just waiting to happen. The less conditioned our musculoskeletal systems are, the higher the chances of injury. Further, it has been shown that the intensity of activity required by a sedentary person trying to improve cardiorespiratory fitness might put that person into a state of excessive overload[52].

Being functional also requires us to challenge our muscles in a proprioceptive enriched environment—**an environment that challenges the internal balance and stabilization mechanisms of the body**.

You see, our muscular system is divided into **prime movers** (thigh, pecs, lats, etc.) and **stabilizers** (erector spinae, transverse abdominis). Prime movers create movement, whereas stabilizers, as the name implies, have more to do with stabilizing your body than creating movement.

In most training programs, stabilizers are not worked, as most exercises are performed on machines. In FBX, you are working out with free weights and dumbbells 100 percent of the time, so your stabilizers are worked to the T. Even then, I would highly recommend giving your stabilizers a really good workout by performing the exercises I have mentioned below.

Exercise to build overall flexibility

Ideally a flexibility session should be performed three times per week immediately after your workout session when your muscles are already warmed up. Flexibility training must be done with a multi-faceted approach that integrates various flexibility techniques in order to achieve optimum soft tissue extensibility in all planes of motion (remember chapter 5 on functional fitness where we discussed the three planes of motions: the sagittal, frontal, and transverse planes).

The following protocols will build overall flexibility

1. **Foam rolling:** This is a technique where muscles are rolled over a cylindrical piece of foam (foam roll) using body pressure to massage micro-adhesions (or knots) in the fibrous tissue that surrounds and supports muscle tissue. It can be used as a cool down process before static stretches.

2. **Static stretching:** This is a process of passively taking a muscle to the point of tension and holding the stretch for a minimum of 20 seconds. It is used to correct muscle imbalances. Static stretching is performed after a workout session.

3. **Active stretching:** In this process, agonists and synergists are used to dynamically move the joint into a range of motion. Active-isolated stretches are suggested for pre-activity warmup. Typically 5 – 10 repetitions of each stretch are performed holding the muscles for 2 – 4 seconds. Active stretching can be performed in between workout sets as well.

List of Stretches
1. Gastrocnemius stretch

2. Soleus stretch

3. Hamstring stretch

4. Standing hip flexor stretch

5. Standing adductor stretch

6. Erector spinae stretch

7. Latissimus dorsi ball stretch

8. Pectoral ball stretch

9. Neck Stretch

Note: How to use a foam roller can be learned by checking out this link: www.bodybuilding.com/exercises/finder/lookup/filter/equipment/id/14/equipment/foam-roll

To improve one's proprioception (balance)

1. Single leg squat

2. Seated Swiss Ball shoulder press

3. Single leg bicep curl

4. Swiss Ball pushups (with variations)

5. Single leg dumbbell row

Note: If you are a hatha yoga lover like me, you can skip these balance exercises as yoga is good enough to work your stabilizers.

To condition your muscles in frontal and transverse planes of motion

Frontal Plane

1. Dumbbell side lunge

2. Dumbbell lateral raise

Transverse plane

1. Wood chop with dumbbell or cable
2. Rotational deadlift to press
3. Dumbbell internal/external rotation

Note: These exercises can be included occasionally in your workouts. You would need to reduce the amount of weight as the idea is to focus on the proprioception component and not on increasing strength.

CHAPTER 15:
FOUR WAYS TO MAKE SURE YOU GET THE BEST WORKOUT EVERY TIME YOU GO TO THE GYM

We all are unique and prefer different settings when it comes to a place to work out. For example, my wife prefers big gyms (the bigger the better), high ceilings, fancy equipment, and a variety of group class offerings. I prefer a rather intimate setting—the ideal scenario would be more like a home gym, with a separate weight room with ample light and very few people if any.

Now, if you have a home gym, rejoice. You will not face the issues I am going to discuss now, but for most of us, a home gym is an expensive proposition, although in the long term it can more than compensate for the money you spend on expensive gym memberships, traveling costs, etc.

But let's face it, the majority of us go to the gym for various reasons, and working out is just one of them. We are social beings, and working on your fitness goals with people around can be a highly stimulating and motivating experience.

My point is that going to a commercial gym has benefits, but the same challenges between an average workout and your personal best come into play. So if you prefer a commercial gym setting to a private fitness studio (or a home gym), following these four important pointers will ensure you a superhero workout every time:

1. **Choose your gym wisely**. There are many considerations when you choose a gym, beginning with location. How far it is from your house, and how much traffic are you likely to encounter on the way? In my experience, traveling for more than 15 – 20 minutes to your gym will test your fitness resolve. Make sure your gym is as close to your house as possible, or better yet, if you commute to work, the gym should lie between your workplace and your home.

Besides the location look at the **equipment and group class offerings. With FBX workouts**, we need simple equipments—a power rack (or a squat rack) to perform squats and a parallel grip bar for deadlifts (most gyms won't have it, and you may have to purchase your own). Also make sure the dumbbells go up to at least 100 pounds so you can vary your workouts with most of the barbell exercises. Since cross training is highly encouraged in FBX, look for a gym that also offers group classes like yoga, spinning, and other body conditioning classes, although they are not a necessity, as HIIT, yoga, etc., can be done in the comfort of your home (or out in the open).

2. **Work out during off-peak times**. Most gyms are crowded during the following times: 7 am to 9 am and 7 pm to 9 pm. Working out at times other than these can be really beneficial so you can concentrate and focus more on your workouts. One major advantage with FBX workouts is that you will spend most of your time near the power rack/squat rack, which usually are the least crowded pieces of equipment, so you generally won't have to wait for your turn, sometimes even during peak hours.

3. **Use headphones for music.** Progressive weight training is concentrated work, and we will have only around three hours a week to make the most of our workouts. Make sure you protect this time fiercely. Ideally, completely shut the outside world out at least a half hour before your workout.

Start by putting your phone on silent, or better, on voicemail. Look at entries from the previous weight session, and enter the weight rooms with a firm goal in mind; know in advance the amount of weight you will lift for a specific exercise and the number of reps you will attempt. Nothing else should matter or put you off track.

Most people in a commercial gym are too distracted with loud pop music blasting throughout the gym, unsympathetic people hogging the equipment and grunting their way on every exercise, and skimpily-dressed women posing as a major distraction. With all this, it becomes nearly impossible to have a good workout. You are guaranteed to complete your sets far below what you are capable of.

Your mind is the ultimate weapon, and trust me when I say that you are much stronger than you allow yourself to be in the gym. With your personal selection of music playing in your headphones, you will zone out and definitely lift more weight than you otherwise would. If you feel the need to socialize, finish your workout and hang out near the juice bar while enjoying a delicious post-workout drink!

4. **Have the courage to do what is right**. Commercial gyms, like Fitness First, 24 Hour Fitness, etc. are places where everyone is doing split routines or spending most of their time in the cardio section. Chances will be very high that you will be the odd one out with the abbreviated routine style discussed in this book. You may feel self-conscious, especially if you are a beginner/intermediate. You will encounter the naysayers, the gigglers, and/or get a lot of free advice from "know it all" dudes on what you should or should not do.

NEVER MIND THEM. SIMPLY IGNORE THEM, or just smile, nod, and keep doing your thing. Most of them have no clue of what they are doing. They are the insecure lot and are probably more self-conscious than you are!

In the end, the mentality (standard split routines, isolation exercises, excessive use of supplements) of a commercial gym environment is quite different from what I advocate. Over time, you should try to find a place where using an abbreviated style of training is the norm, or better yet, arrange to set up a home/garage gym where your mind can be completely free from all the distractions discussed above. If you don't like training alone, find a training partner or two, and you'll be set.

Now, this chapter would be incomplete without a discussion of the gym etiquette one should follow at all times (sort of like a code of conduct for weightlifters). I call this paying tribute and respect to the iron game, and it is part of being inspirational—the third pillar of Fabulous Body (the topic for the last chapter). I know most of you are already following most, if not all, the rules, but this comprehensive list is nothing short of amazing, and I urge you to have a look be sure you are not missing anything: www.bretcontreras.com/-50-commandments-commercial-gym-etiquette/. Points 30, 49, and 50 are my favorites.

SECTION 3:
NUTRITION:
THE REALITY DIET

CHAPTER 16:
FOUR KEY NUTRITIONAL HABITS THAT YOU SHOULD DEVELOP

Every day some new research in the field of nutrition promises better health and more energy. Of course with all this new research there is more opportunity to make better choices. However the sheer volume of information and data can be confusing and overwhelming.

In trying to decide what to take from all of the nutrition advice out there, a good start is:

1. Cut down the refined stuff: white bread, white rice, refined sugars, etc.
2. Eat more vegetables and fruits.
3. Stop eating processed food.
4. Eat more whole foods.

These are basic guidelines that you will hear from most fitness professionals and dietitians.

Now, I will give you something that you can really sink your teeth into.

I don't believe in diets. Fad diets (Atkins, the Zone Diet, etc.) have an element or two that is healthy, but they always miss the bigger picture. Most of fad diets are too restrictive (often requiring you to eliminate an entire macronutrient like carbohydrates or fat), and they rely on a rather regimented and strict approach to eating.

Did you know that more than 95 percent of dieters who lose weight on a diet gain it back[53]?

Instead we will apply timeless holistic principles to nutrition. If you get them right, you can eat all the food you love (yes that cheesecake also) and still keep fat off and build the lean physique you so deserve.

I don't endorse six-pack abs. I am not literally against them, but they are a small part of the whole story of fitness and health. The problem with an extremely ripped look (body fat less than 9 percent) is that it leads to an obsessive lifestyle. What I propose is practical and balanced approach to life and fitness, and if that gives me abs that's fine.

It's not just what you eat, it's also what gets in the way to tempt you.

If I am going out with my family, and I'm tempted to have a full cream latte with cheesecake, I will have it without feeling guilty. Again, the first law of fabulous body applies—eat healthy 80 percent of the time and 20 percent of the time you can eat whatever you want (of course in limits)

The holistic guidelines I'm about to describe are easy to follow. At first there will be some work to develop them into habits, but once you do, good health will be yours. These guidelines are not a one-off thing that you follow for few months until you reach your ideal weight and then resort back to your old lifestyle. You'll need to implement them until they become second nature. This is the easiest "diet" you will have followed yet. I promise you will get the best results.

As I've mentioned again and again, it's never easy to build that lean body, but as you read in the Mindset section of this book, if you are looking for a quick fix, I cannot help you. You must give your body enough time to adapt to a stimulus. Meanwhile, love the way you look right now and start working towards a better you.

Let's start by building four key nutritional habits that over time will help you build a lean, fit and healthy physique:

Key nutritional habit number #1: Start measuring the food you eat.

One excellent approach to good nutrition is creating a food diary to keep track of the food items you eat on a daily basis. Having an **approximate** idea of how many calories you are ingesting can be a huge help in reaching your goal.

Buy a food scale and weigh your food before you eat it. You can find the caloric content of food pretty easily by googling it, and this will give you a clear idea of how many calories you're eating. Most people are surprised to see just how few different foods they actually consume on a daily basis.

For example, for the past five years, whole eggs have been a staple breakfast for me at least five times a week. Add nuts, a portion of meat, dairy products (milk, yogurt), and some fruits, and that's almost 80 percent of my calorie intake for the day. My total ingredient list contains no more than 20 items!

In addition to measuring your food another important approach is eating mindfully and slowly (Fabulous Body Law #4). It takes around 15 minutes for your body to inform your brain that you are full, so be sure to wait at least that long before deciding if you want a second helping. If you tend to have a second serving when the food is delicious (as I often do), use a smaller plate, and make sure you don't overload it the first time. Find what works for you and do it!

Key nutritional habit number #2: Always plan ahead

Planning your meals ahead of time is essential if you want to implement healthy eating habits. I advocate a very practical approach that entails eating just two or three meals a day as opposed to five or six smaller meals. Go to the grocery store twice a week, or simply delegate this task. There are hundreds of online grocers that can deliver anything you want right to your doorstep. If you don't find any eggs in your fridge in the morning, it's probably because of poor planning on your part. Don't be surprised if you end up eating pancakes and waffles as a result, which then spirals into bad eating throughout the day.

Key nutritional habit number #3: Eat homemade food most of the time.

Once you get into the habit of keeping your fridge stocked with all kinds of healthy foods, decide who in your household will cook and how often. Whether you cook all your meals or delegate cooking to your partner or even a private chef, you will likely be spending more time in your kitchen.

Recently, I went to a restaurant with my wife and had the most amazing sole and green salad. The sole was simply done (the way I like it, with minimal gravy) and the salad had just the right amount of dressing. Even my wife agreed that her barbecue grilled chicken was one of the best she ever had. We asked to speak to the chef to complement him, and we gave him a big tip. One other brilliant thing I did was offer to pay him an hourly sum to come to my home every week and teach me how he made the dish we had at his restaurant and other delicious meals. He was absolutely delighted. Now after 10 sessions, I feel like a real chef, and my home cooking has dramatically improved.

The bottom line is if you want you and your family to stay healthy, you have to eat homemade meals, and since most of us cannot afford the services of a private chef, it's a good idea to invest some time in learning how to cook healthy, delicious meals. **You'll be surprised how easy it is. I have listed some of my favorite meals in the meal section.**

Key nutritional habit number #4: Avoid (or greatly limit) any food that is processed.

Losing weight and building muscles boils down to good clean eating most of the time. But it's actually not what you eat, but what gets in the way to tempt you that is the real problem. A trip to a supermarket will open you to so many distractions that the willpower to eat clean food may easily take a back seat. Initially it's tough not to eat junk because our taste buds have been altered by our habit of eating junk food[54], but then once you start to minimize eating processed foods and replace them with healthy foods, your taste buds will start to cherish real food. When this happens, you will realize how sweet an apple can taste!

Trust me; **once you have developed enough momentum eating good healthy nutritious food, it's tough to go back to the junk.** You just need to get started and build the key habits I have discussed.

Now let's briefly discuss the macronutrients in our diet: fats, proteins and carbs.

CHAPTER 17:
FAT: THE MOST MISUNDERSTOOD MACRONUTRIENT

When most people hear the word "fat," they tend to associate it with the adipose tissue in their bodies. This isn't the only misconception about dietary fat; many people think that vegetable oils are healthy because they have the word "vegetable" in their name.

Fat can be your best friend or your worst enemy. It is easy to get confused when talking about fats because some are good and some are bad. This section will answer the following fat-related questions:

What exactly is fat?
What are the different types of fat?
Which fats are good and which are bad? (The answer might surprise you!)
How many calories should I consume every day from fat sources?

What is fat?

Fats are made of collections of molecules called triglycerides. If this collection is liquid at room temperature, it can be called an oil; if it's solid, it is referred to as a fat. A triglyceride is formed from three fatty acids attached to a glycerol molecule.

What types of fats and oils are there?

Saturated fats are triglycerides that contain only single covalent bonds between fatty acid carbon atoms. Because they lack double bonds, each carbon atom is saturated with hydrogen atoms. A few examples are cocoa butter, palm oil, coconut oil, and red meat.

Not all saturated fatty acids are the same. Their length is what sets the various types apart. The shorter ones, which have a chain length of 3 – 12 carbons, are known as **short-chain saturated fatty acids** and are used by the body for energy.

Medium-chain saturated fatty acids are found in several different foods. Medium-chain triglyceride (MCT) oils are used in special medical formulas for people who need energy from fat but cannot absorb the longer-chain fatty acids. The complete set of medium-chain fatty acids are especially important in infant formulas to duplicate the medium-chain saturated fatty acids found in human breast milk, especially the 12-carbon saturated fatty acid known as lauric acid, which functions as a special antimicrobial (antiviral, antibacterial, and antiprotozoal) fatty acid in human milk. Some good examples of medium-chain saturated fatty acids are coconut oil and palm kernel oil.

These short- and medium-chain saturated fatty acids are NOT deposited to any extent in the adipose tissue.

The long-chain saturated fatty acids range from 14 – 14 carbons. Palmitic acid, with 16 carbons, and stearic acid, with 18 carbons, are the most common saturated fatty acids found in food. The very long-chain saturated fatty acids (ranging from 20 – 24 carbons) are membrane fatty acids, which can be found in the brain.

Monounsaturated fats contain fatty acids with one double covalent bond between two fatty acid carbon atoms. They are not completely saturated with hydrogen atoms. This type of fat can be found in carbon lengths of 14, 16, 18, 20, 22, and 24, but the 18-carbon monounsaturated oleic acid is by far the most common variant. The best-known source of oleic acid is olive oil.

Polyunsaturated fats contain more than one double covalent bond between fatty acid carbon atoms. Polyunsaturated fatty acids are found in lengths of 18, 20 and 22 carbons. The best known fats in this category are omega-6 fatty acids (linoleic, gamma-linolenic, and arachidonic acids) and omega-3 fatty acids (alpha-linolenic, eicosapentaenoic [EPA], and docosahexaenoic [DHA] acids).

All fats and oils, regardless of whether they are of vegetable or animal origin, are some combination of saturated fatty acids, monounsaturated fatty acids, and polyunsaturated linoleic acid and linolenic acid. In general, animal fats such as butter, lard, and tallow contain about 40 – 60 percent saturated fat and are solid at room temperature.

Good Fats

Saturated fats: Saturated fats have gotten a lot of attention in the press over the years, but these fats have been unfairly demonized. It all started with Ancel Keys and the Seven Countries Study. Keys launched the Seven Countries Study in 1958 to research the relationship between dietary patterns and the prevalence of coronary heart disease. He uncovered a direct link between heart disease from high total serum cholesterol and saturated fat intake[55].

However, the study was seriously flawed; Keys started out with data from 22 countries and simply omitted the data from the countries that didn't fit with his hypothesis! For the last four decades, because of him and his deceptive study, we have been eating cereals with skim milk instead of whole egg omelets made in butter.

In 2010, a meta-analysis involving more than 300,000 individuals found no significant evidence that dietary saturated fat is associated with an increased risk of coronary heart disease or cardiovascular disease[56].

A recent article in the *British Medical Journal* by British cardiologist Aseem Malhotra, an interventional cardiology specialist registrar at Croydon University Hospital in London, states[57]:

The mantra that saturated fat must be removed to reduce the risk of cardiovascular disease has dominated dietary advice and guidelines for almost four decades. Yet scientific evidence shows that this advice has, paradoxically, increased our cardiovascular risks. The aspect of dietary saturated fat that is believed to have the greatest influence on cardiovascular risk is elevated concentrations of low density lipoprotein (LDL) cholesterol.

*Yet the reduction in LDL cholesterol from reducing saturated fat intake seems to be specific to large, buoyant (type A) LDL particles, when in fact **it is the small, dense (type B) particles (responsive to carbohydrate intake) that are implicated in cardiovascular disease.***

*Indeed, recent prospective cohort studies have not supported any significant association between saturated fat intake and cardiovascular risk. Instead, **saturated fat has been found to be protective**.*

A meta-analysis of observational studies and 27 randomized, controlled trials published in the *Annals of Internal Medicine* also concluded that current evidence does not clearly support cardiovascular guidelines that encourage high consumption of polyunsaturated fatty acids and low consumption of total saturated fats. This particular analysis included data from more than 600,000 people in 18 countries[58].

Omega-3 fatty acids: The University of Maryland Medical Center states that omega-3 fatty acids reduce inflammation[59] and might help lower the risk of chronic diseases such as heart disease[60] cancer, and arthritis. Omega-3 fatty acids are highly concentrated in the brain and appear to be important for cognitive and behavioral function, such as brain performance and memory[61,62,63],

In fact, infants who do not get enough omega-3 fatty acids from their mothers during pregnancy are at risk of developing vision and nerve problems. Symptoms of omega-3 fatty acid deficiency include fatigue, poor memory, dry skin, heart problems, mood swings, depression, and poor circulation[64,65,66].

Your body cannot make these fatty acids, which is why they are called "essential." We must obtain our essential fatty acids, or EFAs, from the foods we eat.

Bad fats

Polyunsaturated fats: Consider an excerpt from the Weston Price Foundation:

The public has been fed a great deal of misinformation about the relative virtues of saturated fats versus polyunsaturated oils. Politically correct dietary gurus tell us that the polyunsaturated oils are good for us and that the saturated fats cause cancer and heart disease. The result is that fundamental changes have occurred in the Western diet. At the turn of the century, most of the fatty acids in the diet were either saturated or monounsaturated, primarily from butter, lard, tallows, coconut oil, and small amounts of olive oil. Today most of the fats in the diet are polyunsaturated from vegetable oils derived mostly from soy, as well as from corn, safflower, and canola.

Modern diets can contain as much as 30 percent of calories as polyunsaturated oils, but scientific research indicates that this amount is far too high. The best evidence indicates that our intake of polyunsaturates should not be much greater than 4 percent of the caloric total, in approximate proportions of 1 1/2 percent omega-3 linolenic acid and 2 1/2 percent omega-6 linoleic acid.

Excess consumption of polyunsaturated oils has been shown to contribute to a large number of disease conditions including increased cancer and heart disease; immune system dysfunction; damage to the liver, reproductive organs and lungs; digestive disorders; depressed learning ability; impaired growth; and weight gain.

One reason the polyunsaturates cause so many health problems is that they tend to become oxidized or rancid when subjected to heat, oxygen and moisture as in cooking and processing. Rancid oils are characterized by free radicals—that is, single atoms or clusters with an unpaired electron in an outer orbit. These compounds are extremely reactive chemically. They have been characterized as "marauders" in the body for they attack cell membranes and red blood cells and cause damage in DNA/RNA strands, thus triggering mutations in tissue, blood vessels and skin. Free radical damage to the skin causes wrinkles and premature aging; free radical damage to the tissues and organs sets the stage for tumors; free radical damage in the blood vessels initiates the buildup of plaque. Is it any wonder that tests and studies have repeatedly shown a high correlation between cancer and heart disease with the consumption of polyunsaturates? New evidence links exposure to free radicals with premature aging, with autoimmune diseases such as arthritis and with Parkinson's disease, Lou Gehrig's disease, Alzheimer's and cataracts.

Trans fats: Trans fats are created when polyunsaturated vegetable oils are heated in the presence of hydrogen gas in order to make them solidify. Trans fats are used abundantly in processed foods because they improve taste, increase shelf life, and have a less greasy feel. The American Heart Association advises that people avoid consuming products that contain this type of fat.

Trans fats are known to increase blood levels of low-density lipoprotein (LDL), or bad cholesterol, while lowering levels of high-density lipoprotein (HDL), or good cholesterol. Trans fats have also been linked to an increased risk of heart disease and diabetes[67].

Dr. Mary G. Enig, an expert in lipid biochemistry, determined that ingesting trans fats alters the activities of the enzyme system, making it easier to get cancer and harder for prescription drugs to fight it.

Key points on fat and how much to eat from healthy fat sources

I hope I have shown you exactly why you should not fear good fats. Armed with knowledge of which fats are good and which are dangerous, you can approach this macronutrient in the healthiest way possible. This means consuming at least 30 percent of calories from fat for optimal health and for a host of other important functions like the fact that healthy fats are needed for the absorption of fat-soluble vitamins, such as Vitamins A, D, E, and K.

Also keep in mind that fat is digested slowly. This has a magical effect on weight loss because it curbs hunger pangs that tend to lead to overeating carbohydrates, especially the dangerous refined variety.

Do not fear whole milk and whole eggs. Embrace them, and eat them as nature intended.

Do not fear saturated fats. They are your best friends and should be responsible for the majority of the calories you eat from fat.

Avoid trans fats at all costs; they are the worst kinds of fat and wreak havoc on your body.

Be sure to include sources of EFA omega-3, as the body cannot manufacture it. Some good sources include fatty wild-caught fish, flaxseed, and krill oil supplements.

You should absolutely limit your intake of omega-6 polyunsaturated fatty acids (PUFA's) from the majority of vegetable oils. This will improve your ratio of omega-3 to omega-6 fats. Ideally, you should limit consumption of omega-6 fats (sunflower oil, cottonseed oil, etc.) to just 2 – 3 percent of your daily calories.

Make a point of including some lauric acid in your diet because it has superior health properties. Lauric acid can be found in coconut, coconut oil, and other coconut products.

CHAPTER 18:
PROTEIN: HOW MUCH DO YOU ACTUALLY NEED?

Protein is an essential nutrient for your body. Proteins are the building blocks of body tissue and can also serve as an alternate source of fuel when needed. Your body uses protein for growth and maintenance. Proteins also function as enzymes in membranes and as transport carriers and hormones; their components serve as precursors for nucleic acids, hormones, vitamins, and other integral molecules.

One gram of protein contains four calories, and you can stock up on proteins from both animal sources—meats, dairy products, fish, and eggs—and vegan sources—whole grains, pulses, legumes, and nuts.

Proteins are made up of amino acids, which are like building blocks. There are 20 different amino acids that join together in various combinations to make all types of proteins. Some of these amino acids can't be made by our bodies, hence they are known as *essential* amino acids, because it is *essential* that our diet provide them. In terms of diet, protein sources are categorized according to how many of the essential amino acids they provide.

A **complete** protein source is one that provides all of the essential amino acids. Complete proteins are also referred to as *high quality proteins*. Animal-based food sources such as meat, poultry, fish, milk, eggs, and cheese are complete protein sources.

An *incomplete* protein is one that is low in one or more of the essential amino acids.

Plant-based food sources such as grains, lentils, and rice are incomplete proteins.

Complementary proteins are two or more incomplete protein sources that together provide adequate amounts of all essential amino acids. For example, rice contains low amounts of the amino acid lysine and high amounts of the amino acid methionine; however, dry beans contain greater amounts of lysine and lesser amounts of methionine. Together, these two food sources can provide adequate amounts of all the essential amino acids required by the human body.

Protein Requirements for Sedentary Versus Active Individuals

The main factors that determine how much protein an individual needs are training regime and habitual nutrient intake. At the same time, current literature suggests that it may be too simplistic to rely on current recommendations for daily protein intake. There are various factors that need to be considered, such as the quality of proteins according to the biological value of the source, caloric intake, exercise intensity, duration and type of exercise, training history, gender, age, etc.

Currently, the RDA for protein intake is 0.8 grams per kilogram of bodyweight, which is based on the needs of sedentary individuals; this represents an intake level necessary to replace losses and avert deficiency. However, this recommended intake is not likely to offset the oxidation of protein/amino acids during exercise, nor it is sufficient to provide an increase in lean tissue and repair of exercise-induced muscle damage because RDA guidelines do not reflect the requirements of hard training individuals seeking to increase muscle mass. Numerous studies indicate protein requirements for active individuals are approximately double that of the RDA—at least 1.4 – 2.0 grams per kilogram of bodyweight[68,69,70,71].

Here's an example to illustrate this clearly.

If an individual weighs about 70 kilograms (154 pounds) and his energy intake averages around 2,000 calories per day, his protein requirement depends upon his choice of activity (intensity, duration, and type) and is one of the following:

The International Society of Sports Nutrition suggests that individuals who exercise ingest protein ranging from 1.4 – 2.0 grams/kg/day.

Individuals engaging in **endurance exercise** should ingest levels at the lower end of this range, or 1.4 grams/kg/day. In this case, the person should consume about 70 (bodyweight in kilos) x 1.4 (grams of protein) = 98 grams of protein per day.

Individuals engaging in **intermittent activities,** such as football, rugby, etc., should ingest levels in the middle of this range, or 1.7 grams/kg/day. In this case, the person should consume about 70 (bodyweight in kilos) x 1.7 (grams of protein) = 119 grams of protein per day.

People engaging in **strength/power exercises,** such heavy weight training, should ingest levels at the upper end of this range, or 2 grams/kg/day. In this case, the person should consume about 70 (bodyweight in kilos) x 2 (grams of protein) = 140 grams of protein per day.

A protein intake above 2 grams/kg/day is only advised in special cases, such as very high energy intake. In the above example, if an individual is an athlete and has a caloric requirement of 4,000 calories, then calculating his protein requirement at a modest level of only 12 – 15 percent of the total calories gives us about 150 grams (15 percent of 4,000 calories = 600/4 = 150 grams), which is 2.14 grams/kg/day. However, these cases are very rare, and the lower amounts described above should be sufficient for most recreational athletes.

Protein and the Kidneys

You might be wondering if consuming 1.4 – 2 grams of protein per kilogram of bodyweight will harm your kidneys. The long-term effects of high protein intake on chronic kidney disease are still poorly understood, and there isn't significant evidence which can link a high protein diet with kidney issues[72,73].

A study compared normal healthy adults following a normal, unrestricted protein diet with a group of vegetarians who maintained a long-term low-protein diet. The results suggest that a high protein non-vegetarian diet does not significantly affect how the kidney functions with regards to "normal aging" in healthy subjects[74]. However, if you have renal issues, consult your physician before you embark on a high protein diet.

Protein Recommendations

RDA guidelines for protein intake are less than the amount actually required for active individuals and should thus be adjusted according to one's type of activity as explained above. Aim to consume at least 1.4 grams/kg/day of protein from various foods to get all the essential amino acids. If you are planning to add a protein supplement to your diet, read the chapter on supplementation for more information.

CHAPTER 19:
CARBOHYDRATES: HOW MUCH SHOULD I EAT?

Carbohydrates include sugars, starches, glycogen, and cellulose. Even though they are a large and diverse group of organic compounds with several functions, carbohydrates represents only 2 – 3 percent of your total body mass.

Carbon, hydrogen, and oxygen are the elements found in carbohydrates. The ratio of hydrogen to oxygen atoms in carbohydrates is usually 2:1, the same as in water. Although there are exceptions, carbohydrates generally contain one water molecule for each carbon atom. This is the reason they are called carbohydrates, which means "watered carbon."

The three major groups of carbohydrates, based on size, are **monosaccharides**—glucose (the main blood sugar), fructose (found in fruits), galactose (found in milk), deoxyribose (in DNA), and ribose (in RNA); **disaccharides**—sucrose (glucose+fructose), lactose (glucose+galactose), and maltose (glucose+glucose); and **polysaccharides**—glycogen, the form of carbohydrates stored mainly in liver and skeletal muscles.

How much carbohydrate should I include in my diet?

Carbs and fats are the most hotly debated macronutrients. Paleo diet advocates swear by a low carb approach and suggest it's the best way to optimize health and lose weight. On the other hand, a Mediterranean diet includes a moderate amount of carbs. An Indian diet is pretty high in carbs and can easily reach up to 70 percent carbs in most cases.

So who is right? Let's find out.

Agriculture was developed around 10,000 years ago. Before that, all humans got their food by hunting, gathering, and fishing. According to anthropologists, hunter-gatherers did not get high blood pressure, arteriosclerosis, or cardiovascular disease. The current craze of Paleolithic diets is based on the idea that our genes were developed 2.6 million years ago and haven't adapted to farmed foods (which have only been around for 10,000 years). Paleo advocates suggest eating plenty of lean meat and fish but *not* dairy products, beans, or cereal grains. The idea is basically to avoid foods introduced into our diet after the invention of cooking and agriculture.

But is it really true that we all evolved to eat a meat-centric diet? Not according to Alyssa Crittenden, a nutritional anthropologist at the University of Nevada, Las Vegas, who studies the diet of Tanzania's Hazda people (some of the last true hunter-gatherers who remain on the planet). The Hazda live on what they find: game, honey, and plants, including tubers, berries, and baobab fruit. They get 70 percent of their energy from plants.

From the above discussion, we can conclude that **there is tremendous variation in what foods humans can thrive on.**

Dr. Joseph Mercola has done a wonderful job at figuring out this genetic variation and has developed a set of questionnaires designed to determine a person's nutritional type.

The results classify people as one of three types: **carb type, protein type, or mixed type**. Carb types feel best when most of their food is healthy carbohydrates, whereas protein types operate best on a low carbohydrate, high protein, relatively high fat diet. Mixed types require food combinations somewhere in between the carb and protein type groups.

Dr. Mercola's questionnaire is a free test that anyone can take to figure out what type he or she is and accordingly the kind of diet needed to experience optimal health. Try it. It doesn't take long. Be sure to watch the video first in the link given below. products.mercola.com/nutritional-typing/

A special note on sugar: Is excessive sugar bad for you?

Even if you are a carb type and genetically thrive on a high carb diet (somewhere close to 50 percent or more of your total caloric intake), understand that the type of carbs that were available even 100 years ago are not the same as the ones available today. The majority of the carbs you find today are the refined type.

So the answer to the question of whether sugar is bad for you is yes; sugar is bad if eaten in excess or when eaten in processed, refined, and artificial form.

It's important to eliminate all the refined sugars that have infiltrated our food supply. A basic education in how to read labels and a trip to your commercial supermarket will help you realize that sugar sneaks into almost every food item that is processed, from tomato ketchup (every 100 grams has 22 grams of sugar) to low fat salad dressings to instant soups. Also did you know that in the 1900s, sugar consumption in the U.S. was 90 pounds of sugar per person per year? By 2009, it had risen to a whopping 180 pounds of sugar per person!

Three harmful effects of eating excessive sugar

Harmful effect number #1: Excessive sugar consumption causes obesity.

There is a close parallel between the upsurge in obesity and rising levels of consumption of SSBs (sugar-sweetened beverages). SSBs include soft drinks, fruit drinks, sports drinks, energy and vitamin water drinks, and sweetened iced tea.

Recently, a large number of epidemiological studies quantified the relationship between SSB consumption and long-term weight gain, type 2 diabetes, and cardiovascular diseases risk[75].

In a meta-analysis of 88 studies, a clear association among soft drink intake, increased energy intake, and body weight was found. Higher soft drink intake was also associated with lower intakes of milk and calcium, as well as lower intakes and other nutrients and an increased risk of several medical problems, including diabetes[76,77].

Harmful effect number #2: Excessive sugar consumption can cause type 2 diabetes.

If one starts to eat too much sugar, a metabolic syndrome called insulin resistance can develop. In this case, your pancreas releases more insulin to curb the excess sugar in your blood stream, but eventually it loses the battle. Your blood sugar keeps rising, and you end up with diabetes[78,79].

Harmful effect number #3: Excessive sugar consumption can give you cancer.

There are multiple studies that link higher sugar consumption with cancer[80,81,82].

CHAPTER 20:
CALCULATING MACRONUTRIENT RATIOS AND TOTAL DAILY ENERGY EXPENDITURE

Once you have figured out your nutritional type, you can go ahead and calculate your optimal macronutrient ratio. Start by calculating your protein requirements. In the protein section we figured that it is roughly 1.4 – 2.0 grams/kg of bodyweight. This should be roughly **25 – 30 percent of your total caloric intake.** We will calculate total daily energy expenditure (TDEE) in the next section.

The next step is to figure out fat requirements. We will eat around **25 – 30 percent of calories from fat** as well. If you have been misguided by conventional wisdom to completely cut fat from your diet, 25 – 30 percent may seem overwhelming. Don't worry; gradually work towards reaching this amount. Start eating whole eggs, include different types of nuts in your diet, use coconut oil and/or ghee for cooking, and you will get to the required percentage.

Once we have figured out the percentage of calories we need from proteins and fat, we are left with calories from carbohydrates. **In general, 30 – 50 percent of calories will come from carb sources.**

Start experimenting with your meals according to whether you are a carb type, protein type, or a mixed type. Maintain a diary detailing how you feel after having a high protein diet or a high carb meal. I personally have taken the test repeatedly and have come out to be the **mixed type**. I do well on moderate carbs. I cycle my carbs around my workouts and stay low carb on days when I don't go to the gym.

Consider this table for a person who weighs 75 kg (165 pounds) and has a caloric requirement of 2000 calories per day:

% OF TOTAL CALORIES	LOW (4 – 20%)	MODERATE (20 – 40%)	HIGH (40% +)
CARBS (in grams)	20 – 100	100 – 200	200 +
% IN RELATION TO THE TOTAL CALORIES	LOW (9 – 20%)	MODERATE (20 – 40%)	HIGH (40% +)
FAT (in grams)	20 – 45	45 – 88	88 +
GRAMS PER KG OF BODYWEIGHT	LOW (0.5 – 0.8)	MODERATE (0.8 – 2)	HIGH (2 +)
PROTEIN (in grams)	37.5 – 75	75 – 150	150 +

How to calculate your Total Daily Energy Expenditure (TDEE)

Your TDEE is the number of calories your body burns in a 24-hour period while sleeping, working, exercising, playing, and even digesting food.

TDEE is the sum of BMR + TEA. Let's briefly discuss each of these measurements.

Basal metabolic rate (BMR): This is the number of calories you burn at rest (lying down, watching TV, or working on your laptop). These calories are required for your brain to function and for your heart to beat. Most people's BMR is about 60 – 75 percent of their TDEE depending on their activity levels.

Thermic effect of activity (TEA): The more you move and exercise, the higher your TEA. In addition, the more intense your training session, the more calories you burn overall. That's why weight training burns more calories than a moderate intensity cardio session. Studies show that energy post-oxygen consumption (EPOC) following a period of intense heavy resistance training elevates the metabolism for as long as 24 hours following the resistance session.

There are various formulas for estimating your BMR and total caloric expenditure. Let's look at the two most popular ones.

The Katch-McArdle Equation

BMR = 370 + (9.79759519 x lean mass in pounds)

The Mifflin-St Jeor Equation

For men: BMR = 10 x weight (kg) + 6.25 x height (cm) – 5 x age (years) + 5

For women: BMR = 10 x weight (kg) + 6.25 x height (cm) – 5 x age (years) – 161

Once you have determined your BMR, you need to multiply it by the appropriate activity factor to determine your total daily caloric needs. The factors are:

1.200 = sedentary (little or no exercise)

1.375 = light activity (light exercise/sports 1 – 3 days/week)

1.550 = moderate activity (moderate exercise/sports 3 – 5 days/week)

1.725 = very active (hard exercise/sports 6 – 7 days/week)

1.900 = extra active (very hard exercise/sports and a physically demanding job)

If you're having trouble deciding between two activity factors, choose the lower one to be on the safe side.

CALORIC REQUIREMENTS FOR WEIGHT LOSS

15 percent below maintenance: This is a conservative deficit and a slow way to lose fat. If there are no deadlines and you need to retain maximum lean muscle mass, this is the best estimate.

20 percent below maintenance: This is a moderate deficit for people who have above average body fat levels.

25 percent below maintenance: This is an aggressive plan to lose fat and can be used for a short period of time for people who have significant body fat stores.

CALORIC REQUIREMENTS FOR WEIGHT GAIN

15 percent above maintenance: This is a slow way to gain weight and suitable when the goal is a conservative increase. If there are no deadlines and you need to make sure that you don't gain too much fat, this is the best estimate.

20 percent above maintenance: This is a moderate increase for people who have some trouble gaining weight.

25 percent above maintenance: This is an aggressive plan to gain weight and can be used for a short period of time.

Let's take an example to put everything in perspective.

Sally is 30 years old, weighs 140 pounds, has 30 percent body fat, and is 160 cm (5' 3") tall. She has a sedentary job and her only activity is going to the gym a few times per week.

To calculate her lean mass: Sally's fat mass is 0.3*140 = 42 pounds. Therefore, her lean mass is 140 − 42 = 98 pounds.

Using the formulas for calculating caloric expenditure, we can plug in Sally's numbers to find out how many calories she needs per day to maintain her current weight.

Using the Katch-McArdle Equation

BMR = 370 + (9.79759519 x Lean Mass in pounds) = 370 + (9.7975 * 98) = 1329.42

TDEE = 1329.42 * 1.55 TEA = **2059**

Using the Mifflin-St. Jeor Equation

Female BMR = 10 x weight (kg) + 6.25 x height (cm) − 5 x age (years) − 161 = 10 * 63.63 + 6.25* 160 — 5* 30 —161 = 1322

TDEE = 1322 * 1.55 TEA = **2049.**

CHAPTER 21:
INTERMITTENT FASTING: A SUPERIOR WAY TO EAT?

True or False?

1. Breakfast is the most important meal of the day.

2. I need to eat five to six smaller meals throughout the day if I want to lose weight.

3. I need to ingest protein every three to four hours to avoid muscle breakdown.

These statements are what conventional wisdom dictates to be true. Do they work? Maybe, but what if I tell you there is better way to eat that will not only save you time, but will make you stronger, leaner, and healthier at the same time.

Interested? I bet you are.

So what is intermittent fasting and how can it help you build a lean, sexy, healthy physique and in the process save lots of time and effort?

IF is not starvation!

Starvation is restricting calories severely to fewer than 1000 per day in order to lose weight quickly. **Intermittent fasting is about decreasing the frequency of meals while keeping the required number of calories intact.** Essentially what it means is that instead of eating, say, 2000 calories over five to six smaller meals throughout the day you'll be eating three or even two meals a day (sometimes just one).

Fasting for more than 24 hours is something I have not done. However, the benefits of prolonged fasting on health are significant, and there is enough evidence to support that it does more good than harm.

As I strictly preach what I practice, in this section I will only discuss two types of eating patterns (limited to a 24-hour period only) that I have been following for the past year and half.

One meal a day

This type of meal plan is comprehensively explored in Ori Hofmekler's fascinating book, *The Warrior Diet*. The gist of the Warrior Diet is to eat only one meal a day, preferably at night, without any restriction of calories or macronutrient content. During the day, Ori recommends eating fresh vegetables, fruits, and a little protein that doesn't included any carbs like breads or grains.

The Warrior Diet guarantees you several hours a day of fat- hormones burning (read: no insulin) percolating throughout your body. Ori further states that during these hours, your body is at peak capacity to remove toxins and generate energy while staying alert and resisting fatigue and stress. Long periods of undereating **increase protein efficiency**, so when you do eat protein, it will be utilized much more efficiently.

Not eating for long periods also **improves insulin sensitivity,** so when you do eat, your blood sugar doesn't fluctuate wildly, and your body won't store carbohydrate calories as fat.

Eating only one meal a day works perfectly well for me, as I usually research and write my articles in the morning for a few hours when I know my creativity is at its peak. I don't want to stop to cook breakfast, which I know will take away an hour, and who knows if I will feel like writing again after my meal? So I skip breakfast and simply sip water, black coffee, or green tea until lunch.

When lunchtime arrives, if I decide I need to keep working but I am feeling slightly hungry, I have something light like a whey protein shake or boiled eggs, etc., and at the same time, I plan my sumptuous dinner. (Planning the dinner becomes really important as that one meal will decide how healthy you will eat for that day.) This kind of intermittent fasting means eating all of your required calories in one meal, however, you need to build to it slowly. At first, eating this many calories at once can be intimidating and tough for the body to accept.

Also note that during the undereating periods you are allowed to eat light foods that are not taxing on your digestive system, like whey protein, boiled eggs, and tea/coffee without milk or cream. So yes, you do get some calories from these foods.

There are three times I practice this one meal a day pattern of IF:

1. During my off workout days when I work the whole day and don't have time to plan, prepare, and eat meals.
2. When I plan to eat a buffet at my favorite restaurant and I can't help eating over 2000 calories.
3. When I am traveling most of the day and can't get access to good food.

Two or three meals a day

When I follow this as a pattern, I simply skip one of my main meals (usually lunch). I routinely have whole eggs in the morning, as my two-year-old son loves them, and it's a good way to bond with him—a wonderful start to my day. Then I usually skip lunch, as eating in the afternoon makes me sleepy. Skipping lunch also allows me to work productively until early evening and prepare for a sumptuous dinner.

Now, on days when I **work out with weights, I usually eat three square meals**. I opt for a heavy breakfast made of oats, milk, and eggs. I then again have a high carb meal before and after my workout, making sure that I am close to my required calorie range each time.

The best part about IF is you don't have to be hell-bent on doing it a particular way or in a pattern. You can choose whatever way suits your mood and your lifestyle. But if you are looking for a structured approach, Martin Berkhan from Lean Gains does a good job recommending a structured approach. He suggests a 14-hour fast for women and 16-hour fast for men, then "feeding" for the remaining eight to ten hours. So you are fasting the entire night and eating only after five to six hours of being awake. During the feeding window, you can have a few meals to fulfill your required caloric intake.

The only thing you need to ensure is that you eat the same number of calories in each 24-hour period so that your body doesn't slows its metabolism down or start burning down lean muscles.

Other Patterns of IF you can follow for even more flexibility

In his new book, *The Fast Diet*, Dr. Michael Mosley suggests the best way to lose weight is to eat normally for five days a week and fast for two. On fasting days, he recommends cutting down to 25 percent of your normal daily calories or about 600 calories for men and 500 for women, along with plenty of water and tea. He claims to have lost 19 pounds in two months by following this eating pattern.

Brad Pilon, author of *Eat Stop Eat* suggests fasting for 24 hours once or twice a week. After the fast, he says to then go back to eating normally. "Act as if you didn't fast," Pilon says.

The reason this may work is there will be a reduction in total average calories that you eat in a week, which will give your body a break and allow it to heal itself and of course lose fat.

The main reason I practice IF is that it saves me time and effort in planning, cooking, and eating meals. For me, every meal needs to be healthy with the low-moderate carb macronutrients according to my preference (and high carbs around my workouts).

I feel following any kind of diet is restrictive. Your hunger, your lifestyle, and of course your goals should dictate what you do or do not do.

Five awesome health benefits of IF

1. **It saves lots of time and effort.** As you must have figured out, fewer meals means less time planning, preparing, and cooking.

2. **It improves insulin sensitivity.** A limited number of trials have been done on humans, but early results have shown that IF can significantly improve insulin sensitivity[83].

3. **IF helps reduce total caloric intake overall** and therefore can be beneficial to heart health and chronic disease prevention[84,85,86]. Periodic fasting is also

associated with reduction in coronary heart disease[87,88].

4. **It helps you be consistent with your diet plan**. When you have fewer meals to plan, you will tend to stick to your eating schedule better over the long term, which ultimately leads to a leaner, stronger physique. Fasting is no mystery to us humans. Muslims fast during their holy period of Ramadan, Hindus fast for various religious reasons, and we instinctively don't eat when we are sick. Our genetics were built 2.5 million years ago when humans alternated between periods of feast and famine.

5. **Over time you will become more successful**. Although it's pretty hard to quantify, with periods of undereating (or complete fasting), I feel powerful, alert, more aware, relaxed, creative and raring to take on the world. This is when my sympathetic nervous system is dominant. The sympathetic nervous system is the fight or flight system, which promotes alertness and energy expenditure and is mainly catabolic, hence productivity is improved. **With a lighter body and a clear mind I also become more self-aware and grateful for things around me.**

These periods of undereating or fasting are also the times when my insulin levels are the lowest, and of course we know what happens when insulin is low. The body burns fat like crazy. On the other hand, when someone eats, the parasympathetic nervous system becomes dominant. This system is responsible for digestion and sleep. It promotes relaxation and replenishment of energy reserves and is mainly anabolic. That's why people often feel sleepy after eating lunch.

Intermittent patterns of eating work in synergy with both the sympathetic and parasympathetic nervous systems without compromising one or the other.

My not-so-good experience with eating five to six meals a day and my recommendation

I consider myself quite disciplined when it comes to training and eating right. I was willing to eat boiled chicken with broccoli all the time. I was willing to cook all of my day's meals in advance, and I even set an alarm for every three hours to remind me to eat and avoid breakdown of my muscles. I enjoyed the process, as conventional wisdom (top bodybuilders and veteran trainers) convinced me it was the only way to achieve a perfectly lean and sculpted body. I followed through, but then eventually it started to affect me. I started to become obsessed about it. It started to affect my work, as the moment I finished a meal I started thinking about the next one. Worst of all, I hardly saw any results.

With IF, my recommendation is to try out this method slowly. If you are eating five or six meals a day now, cut down to three and then two. The idea is to give your body a break long enough for it to heal itself.

How I Stay On Track With My Diet

Calories and Macronutrients

Depending on my phase (cutting or gaining) and irrespective of the number of meals and shakes I consume daily, I eat the required number of calories in order to lose weight or gain weight. I also make sure that my protein intake is above 150 grams every day. The top foods I eat for protein are whole eggs, cow's milk, and either chicken, fish, or lentils.

I usually eat high carb meals around my workouts to replenish my glycogen stores and provide the required energy for my workouts. I always cook in desi-ghee, and extra virgin coconut oil, and I use extra virgin olive oil to pour over salads and pasta dishes. My intake of oils rich in polyunsaturated fatty acids is close to zero with limited amounts only when I eat out (although I still insist that the chef cook in saturated fats if that option exists).

I eat *slowly and mindfully*, chewing and savoring every bit. I usually start off by eating a salad, then my protein source, and then my carbs (brown rice, chapattis, etc.). The amount of carbs I consume in a day depends on my appetite and my workouts.

I "google" the nutrient content of the foods I eat in order to find out their caloric values. A day in advance, I mentally visualize what I plan to eat the next day and try to stay as close to my required caloric intake as possible. I'm usually aware when I overeat, but I do allow myself a few indulgences now and then, mainly during my gaining phase. For example, sometimes I feel like having few glasses of wine or that New York cheesecake (with the big scoop of vanilla ice cream). When I do eat these things, I step up the intensity of my next workout: it works out very well.

Keeping within my fat range

I don't weigh myself too often. Instead, I rely on how my clothes fit me, and I keep a close eye on my waist. I don't focus on the scale or my body fat levels too much and often view looking at myself in the mirror as the best guide. My waist (measured from my navel) moves between 31 inches when I am leanest to 33 inches. I start to get a bit conscious if it crosses 33 inches, and that's when I make changes in my lifestyle, using diet and exercise to bring it back to less than 33 inches and ideally to 31. This corresponds to anywhere from 10 − 14 percent of body fat. As of now, I have no plans to compete in fitness competitions, and don't see any reason why I should take my fat level below 12 percent. To measure body fat, I use a skin-fold calipers or a body fat bioelectrical machine (usually found in commercial gyms).

Healthy foods are key

Over time, I have made sure my kitchen and fridge are stocked with nutritious foods and my and my family's taste buds have evolved to where we now only eating good, nutritious foods. One of the key habits I have developed is to shop at least once a week for groceries. If you have healthy food in your kitchen, chances become very high that you will eat it.

Including ample protein and enough healthy fats in my meals ensures I don't have cravings at all. There were times when long breaks in between meals were a challenge, but eventually my body adapted. Whenever I feel hungry, I simply snack on something healthy and light or drink water, green tea, or even black coffee to alleviate that craving. Some healthy snack options are juiced vegetables, yogurt with plain almonds, any type of salad, sprouts, a plain glass of cow's milk, coconut water, carrots with hummus/dip, etc.

I don't have any pre-workout snacks; instead, I simply make sure that I have a high complex carb meal two to three hours before my workout with enough quality protein and fats, and I am good to go. I make sure I have a good night's sleep the previous night, have my high carb breakfast and lunch to replenish my glycogen stores and sometimes take a power nap right before my workout. I also have black coffee right before my workout. That's it. I never rely on those expensive chemical-laden pre-workout drinks. After a workout, I have a protein shake with water and a couple of bananas. If I am not hungry right after my workout, I then have a nice sumptuous dinner within few hours.

TABLE 1: MY WEEKLY MEAL PLAN

Time	Monday	Tuesday	Wednesday	Thursday	Friday	Saturday	Sunday
8 – 9 am	Ginger Tea, Then Coffee W/Cookie	Lemon Juice W/Honey, Then English Tea	Wheat Grass Shot, Then Coffee W/Cookie	Lemon Juice W/Honey, Then English Tea	Ginger Tea, Then Coffee W/Cookie	Ginger Tea, Then Coffee W/Cookie	Wheat Grass Shot W/Honey, Then English Tea
9:30 – 10:30 am	Omelet (5 Whole Eggs) Made In Coconut Oil, 2 Slices Multi-Seed Whole Wheat Bread Banana-Cinnamon Oatmeal With Unprocessed Honey	5 Whole Boiled Eggs, 2 Slices Multi-Seed Whole Wheat Bread Big Bowl Of Papaya/ Pineapple	Scrambled Eggs With Vegetables Stirred In Extra Virgin Coconut Oil, 2 Slices Multi-Seed Whole Wheat Bread	Skip	Omelet (5 Whole Eggs) Made In Coconut Oil, 2 Slices Multi-Seed Whole Wheat Bread Banana-Cinnamon Oatmeal With Unprocessed Honey	Banana Grand Whey Smoothie (Banana, Whey, Milk, Flaxseed, 3 Raw Eggs, Honey)	Skip
2 – 3 pm	Brown Rice W/Black Beans	Skip	Oatmeal W/ Walnuts, Mercola Smoothie	Buffet Meal – Easily Over 2000 Calories		Skip	Sunday Brunch: Chicken Tikka Masala W/ Brown Rice & Cooked Eggplant
4 – 4:30 pm	WORKOUT: WEIGHTS		WORKOUT: WEIGHTS		WORKOUT: WEIGHTS		
6 pm	Mercola Smoothie (Banana, Whey, Water)	Mercola Smoothie (Banana, Whey, Water)			Mercola Smoothie (Banana, Whey, Water)		Mercola Smoothie (Banana, Whey, Water)

Time	Monday	Tuesday	Wednesday	Thursday	Friday	Saturday	Sunday
7:30 – 8:30 pm	Penne With Red Sauce And Canned Tuna	Indian Thali (Cowpeas, Cooked Okra, Chapattis And Some White Rice)	Chicken Cacciatore W/ Brown Rice	Skip	Whole Wheat Spaghetti W/Jamie Oliver Pesto Sauce And Canned Tuna, 2 Glasses Red Wine	Order In: Slowly Cooked Whole Herbed Chicken W/ Big Salad, 2 Glasses Red Wine	Leftovers From Brunch Or Tuna Melt With Avocado
11:30 pm	Plain Cow's Milk	Hot Chocolate W/Cow's Milk		Green Tea			Hot Chocolate W/Cow's Milk

TABLE 2: The ingredient list I have been using for past few years or so

Carbohydrates	Proteins	Fats	Herbs/Spices/ Condiments	Fruits/Vegetables
Oatmeal **Whole Grain Multi-seed Bread** **Brown Rice** **Whole Grain Flour** **Whole Wheat French Bread Baguette** **Whole Wheat Penne**	Eggs (free range) Chicken Breast Turkey Fish of Choice Tuna packed in water Yogurt Full Fat Cow's Milk Cottage Cheese Black Beans Cowpeas Lentils Beans Mature Cheddar Cheese Swiss Cheese	Oils Desi-ghee Extra-Virgin Olive Oil Extra Virgin Coconut Oil Nuts Almonds Walnuts Figs Raisins Dates Cashews Seeds Flaxseeds Pumpkin Sesame	Herbs & Spices Basil Oregano Parsley Thyme Mint Celery Cilantro Jaggery Sugar Dark Brown Sugar Salt Ground Cinnamon Black Pepper Condiments Unprocessed Honey Low-fat Canola Mayonnaise Salsa Lime Juice Mustard Maple Syrup Apple Juice Hummus Dips Pesto Sauce Red Wine Vinegar Hot Pepper Sauce Pasta Sauce Thai Sauce	Vegetables Artichokes Asparagus Broccoli Cabbage Carrots Cucumber Green beans Lettuce: Iceberg, Romaine Garlic Avocados Jalapeños Mushrooms Onions Peppers: Red, Yellow, Green Peas Olives Potatoes Okra Eggplant Cauliflower Bitter-guard Spinach Tomatoes Cherry Tomatoes Zucchini Fruits Apples Bananas Oranges Strawberries Honeydew Melon Watermelon Mangoes Pomegranates

CHAPTER 22:
TOP SUPPLEMENTS THAT YOU SHOULD TAKE ALL YEAR AROUND

There are three supplements that I have been consuming for more than a decade on almost a daily basis. As I mentioned before, supplements, as the word suggests, are just supplements to your wholesome diet and not substitutes for anything in it. These supplements will work best only when you also consume a balanced diet.

Whey protein

Whey protein is an excellent functional food, but it is only as good as the source it comes from and the methods used to process it.

Not all whey is created equal

In one report, fifteen protein powders and drinks were tested for levels of arsenic, cadmium, lead, and mercury. Out of these fifteen, three samples were of particular concern, as they tested high for levels of these toxic chemicals. Consider the fact that cadmium accumulates and can damage kidneys. Furthermore, it can take up to twenty years for the body to eliminate even of half the cadmium it absorbs[89]!

Following are **three** critical points to consider when choosing which protein brand you can trust:

1) **Whey protein should come from grass-fed cows.** Your whey powder should come from cows that are grass-fed and graze all year round in natural pastures. Besides being grass-fed, the cows need to be hormone free and healthy overall. How can you find out more about this? Good companies usually mention this on their website. If you don't find the information there, call their customer service and ask.

2) **Whey processing needs to be done at low temperatures to avoid denaturing the native structures of protein**. Most commercial whey products are derived from pasteurized dairy and are heat-processed, which makes the whey acidic and nutritionally deficient. This damages the immuno-supportive micronutrients and amino acids in the whey.

3) **Whey protein supplements should be sweetened naturally.** Most protein supplement companies use artificial sweeteners that are very harmful for your body, including acesulfame-k[90], sucralose[91,92], artificial flavorings, and soy lecithin. They do this to cut costs. Look for companies that use stevia as a natural sweetener.

Whey concentrates, isolates or hydrolysates: which one to go for?

There are three types of whey on the market: **concentrates, isolates, and hydrolysates**.

Whey isolates are 90 – 96 percent pure protein with very little fat, lactose, and mineral content.

Whey concentrates range from 29 – 89 percent pure protein and are most commonly 80 percent protein. They have higher contents of fat, lactose, and minerals.

Hydrolyzed whey proteins are isolates that undergo a hydrolysis process to break the protein down into smaller groups of amino acids, or peptides, which are predigested. They have a very minuscule amount of fat, lactose, and mineral content, and they are the most expensive on the market. I personally find their taste very bitter.

Most protein isolates available are denatured by-products of cheese manufacturing. Isolates that you find on the market are exposed to acid processing and are also deficient in key nutritional cofactors.

One authority whose work I really like is Ori Hofmekler, and in his own words:

"Most commercial whey products are derived from pasteurized dairy and are processed with heat and acid. Many are also artificially sweetened. All of these factors render them completely useless from a health perspective. **Whey isolate is one such inferior product, because when you remove the fat, you actually remove important components of its immunological properties, such as phospholipids, phosphatidylserine and cortisol.** *Additionally, all of the IgG immunoglobulins, which are an excellent source of glutamine and cysteine, are also bound to the fat globule. Fat provides not just calories. In fact, most food rich in healthful fat, including nuts, seeds, chia and almonds are carriers of antioxidants, such as Vitamin E and phytosterols. Dairy also contains lipoic acid, which is a carrier of enzymes and immunoglobulin. Therefore, if you take the fat out you're left with a clearly inferior whey protein."*

"I'm totally against whey isolate," Ori says. "I think it's just the wrong whey."

I always believe in functional and whole foods. For me any food or even a supplement that I ingest needs to be as unprocessed as possible and not denatured. Therefore, whey concentrates win, hands down! It is cheaper than isolates (and hydrolysates), tastes much better (you'd be blown away if you have one of the protein shakes I make from concentrates), and it has more health benefits than the other two sources.

Most people would argue that whey isolates absorb quickly, which helps in recovery, and that gram by gram, it has a lot more protein. Whey isolates, as I mentioned, are 90 – 96 percent protein, whereas a good whey concentrate is around 80 percent protein. That's a difference of roughly 10 – 16 percent.

If we ingest 50 grams of whey powder, that is only a difference of 5 – 7.5 grams. I would rather add slightly more whey concentrate and take advantage of the health benefits it provides. What about the fat content? Again, I don't really worry about a few grams of fat in my protein considering these fats have a host of beneficial properties. And since I recommend a generous fat intake, it hardly makes a difference!

The only reason to use isolates is if you are lactose intolerant. In that case, I know many people who still do well on concentrates, but if you have tried concentrates and ended up with bloating or gastronomical disturbances, go ahead and use isolates. Still, make sure that your isolates manufacturer fulfills the criteria's outlined earlier.

2. Krill oil

Now, we know that excess consumption of polyunsaturated omega-6 fatty acids can create many problems[93,94,95]. Therefore, **it is important to have the proper ratio of**

omega-3 and omega-6 in the diet[96]. Omega-3 fatty acids help reduce inflammation[97] while most omega-6 fatty acids tend to promote inflammation. The typical American diet contains 14 – 25 times more omega-6 fatty acids than omega-3 fatty acids, which many nutritionally-oriented physicians consider to be way too high on the omega-6 side[98].

Dietary sources of omega-3

Typical recommendations are 0.3 – 0.5 grams per day of omega-3 in the form of EPA+DHA and 0.8 – 1.1 grams of alpha-linolenic acid. These recommendations can be fulfilled by following the AHA dietary guidelines of eating two servings of fish per week with an emphasis on fatty fish such as salmon and herring. Plant foods such as flaxseeds and walnuts contain an omega-3 fat called alpha-linolenic acid (ALA). It is easier for fish to convert alpha-linolenic acid from algae and other sea plants into EPA and DHA; humans can only do so to a very limited degree.

Although ALA is not harmful, you'll ideally want to include the animal-based form in your diet as well. Note that fish and seafood are a major source of human exposure to contaminants like methylmercury and polychlorinated biphenyls (PCBs), so one should focus on eating more wild-caught species and not farm raised. For those individuals who do not eat fish, have limited access to a variety of fish, or cannot afford to buy fish regularly, a fish oil supplement should be considered.

Why krill oil is better than fish oil for omega-3 supplementation

Krill—or "okiami" as the Japanese call it—are small, shrimp-like creatures that have been a cherished food source in Asia since the nineteenth century or possibly even earlier. **The antioxidant potency of krill oil is 48 times higher than that of fish oil.** Krill oil also contains astaxanthin, a marine-source flavonoid that creates a special bond with EPA and DHA to allow the direct metabolism of the antioxidants, making them more bioavailable[99].

I have been consuming krill oil on a daily basis for the past many years, and my health has never been better.

3. Multivitamin-mineral

According to the 2010 Dietary Guidelines for Americans, "For the general, healthy population, there is no evidence to support a recommendation for the use of multivitamin/mineral supplements in the primary prevention of chronic disease."

A National Institutes of Health–sponsored State-of-the-Science Conference also concluded that the present evidence is insufficient to recommend either for or against the use of [multivitamins] to prevent chronic disease.

Despite the lack of definitive trial data regarding the benefits of multivitamins in the prevention of chronic disease, including cancer, many men and women take them for precisely this reason. Apparently, multivitamin-mineral (MVM) supplements are the most commonly used supplements in the Unites States, with at least one third of US adults regularly taking them.

Consider these four studies that establish a strong co-relation between **optimal intake of nutrients and chronic diseases**:

1) Recently, the *Journal of the American Medical Association* (JAMA) reversed a long-standing anti-vitamin

stance by publishing two scientific reviews recommending multivitamin supplements for all adults[100].

In the review, the researchers wrote that the North American diet is generally sufficient to prevent overt vitamin deficiency diseases such as pellagra, scurvy, and beriberi. However, they explain, "recent evidence has shown that suboptimal levels of vitamins, even well above those causing deficiency syndromes, are associated with increased risk of chronic diseases including cardiovascular disease, cancer, and osteoporosis." In a clinical commentary, they note that "a large proportion of the general population" has less than optimal intakes of a number of vitamins, exposing them to increased disease risk. In addition, they counsel that "it appears prudent for all adults to take vitamin supplements."

2) In another study of men, daily multivitamin supplementation was associated with a significant reduction in the risk of cancer[101].

3) A study of 9,000 adults in the *Journal of Nutrition* claimed that long-term use of a multivitamin-mineral is associated with reduced risk of cardiovascular disease mortality among women[102].

4) As stated early in this book, more than a billion people worldwide are Vitamin D deficient. A study published by Garland CF, et. al., concluded that raising the minimum year round serum levels of Vitamin D from 25 ng/ml to 40 – 60 ng/ml would prevent approximately 58,000 new cases of breast cancer and 49,000 new cases of colorectal cancer each year! Such intakes are also expected to reduce case-fatality rates of patients who have breast, colorectal, or prostate cancer by half[103].

The best way to get more Vitamin D is moderate exposure to sun during appropriate times, but with increased time indoors, it's increasingly difficult for us to get the optimal amount from the sun. Getting enough Vitamin D from food is also very difficult. Therefore it becomes essential to take a multivitamin-mineral that has Vitamin D3 in it.

I personally have been taking a multivitamin-mineral supplement for over a decade now even though my diet is pretty healthy, at least that's what I think. Note, though, that due to mass food production, excess processing, and high flame cooking, our foods are less nutrient-dense than before. Even if you eat 5 – 7 servings of fruits and vegetables daily (the majority of us don't), the optimal intake to prevent diseases is much more than the RDAs, and to my knowledge, taking a daily multivitamin-mineral supplement is the best insurance policy. Worried about toxicity or even deaths from supplement use? There is absolutely none[104].

BE INSPIRATIONAL, CONTRIBUTE, GIVE BACK: FOUR FABULOUS WAYS TO DO SO

A fabulous body is inspirational in itself. It is pleasing to look at and not overly ripped or extremely shredded. It looks real and is healthy. If you build one, you will naturally inspire people.

However you can take being an inspiration one step further and pursue it actively.

Fortunately for me, what started as a hobby of helping people to achieve their health and fitness goals became a full-time career. Over the past decade in the fitness industry, I have personally coached and trained hundreds of people and thousands and thousands more have enrolled in my health club to get fit since 2010.

I feel empowered when people come up to me and say, "Because of you, Akash, my life changed." This gives me courage to keep doing what I am doing and reaching out to more and more people. And that's one of the MAIN REASON I wrote this book (and at the same time launched my blog, fabulousbody.com) to potentially reach millions and millions out there who suffer from conventional wisdom. I want to tell them there is a better, more efficient and effective way to reach their health and fitness goals.

Besides this, I have committed 10 percent of net income from Fabulous Body, Inc. to various charitable causes I believe in. I got inspiration from reading about Richard Reed, founder of Innocent Smoothie. He believes that our world would be a very different place if all businesses take 10 percent of their net income and allocate it to people and to countries who need it more than we do, this way it would redistribute wealth while absolutely protecting the capitalist system that we find to be the best way of working.

My motto is quite simple: *Start small and think big.* Most people usually say they don't feel like contributing. They rationalize by saying they will start contributing and giving back only after they have earned x amount of money or when they retire. What I feel is that for most, that time never comes, and therefore I am asking you to start now.

You don't need to start a charity or donate thousands of dollars. You can start very small and eventually build upon that.

Don't know where to start? Here are four awesome ways you can start giving back:

1. **Spread awareness about Vitamin D deficiency.** I have mentioned Vitamin D deficiency a few times in this book, and I want to mention it again, as lack of Vitamin D is linked with various preventable diseases, such as cancer. Through this book and through my blog, I want to spread awareness of the importance of this essential vitamin and the significant role it plays in our body. The first thing you can do is download the Vitamin D app "D-minder" and start measuring your Vitamin D levels. Get yourself checked at a local health clinic or order a test from grassrootshealth.net if you are from United States. As quoted on this site: With only 100 people joining today and getting two friends to join in two weeks (and those two friends getting two more to join), by week 42, there could be 400,000,000 people who are Vitamin D "replete" (more than the United

States population)! With more than a billion people deficient, I think it's becoming a silent epidemic worldwide and requires serious attention.

2. **Donate blood.** Blood cannot be manufactured. It is in constant demand for patients who are battling chronic diseases like cancer. It is required for surgeries and for anyone who has met with an accident. Blood has a short shelf life and therefore is in constant need. Did you know that when you donate blood you are potentially saving three lives? A man can easily give blood four times a year, and a women can give three times yearly. Once you start donating, chances are extremely high that you will become a regular donor. Giving blood doesn't take much of your time. Contact your nearest blood bank and incorporate this wonderful habit into your lifestyle.

3. **Donate money.** With the power of technology and the internet, you can choose any cause and select any charity that matches your interest and passion anywhere in the world and donate in less than a minute. You can start with a bare minimum and build over time.

4. **Gift this book to five people you know who would benefit from reading it.** However, do this only after you have gotten good results from following the suggestions and recommendations I have given and firmly believe that the information could bring about a change to their lives.

Don't feel like contributing or giving back? Well....MEDITATE.

As Swami Vivekananda puts it, **"Meditation is everything."** Our planet needs a shift of consciousness. Meditation, we all know, is a higher state of consciousness. The Dalai Lama once said, "If every eight year old in the world is taught mediation, we will eliminate violence from the world within one generation."

Such an empowering quote. When we meditate, we become mindful of things around us. We start to think more clearly and appreciate the simpler things in life. Meditation allows us to be grateful for things, and once you are grateful, you start to operate from a different mindset of total abundance and unconditional love. You can't help but give back and contribute.

This part slowly sank in with me. A few years back, if you'd ask me to give blood, I would have walked the other way. But recently, I organized a blood camp at my health club, and I knew potentially hundreds of lives were saved because of the initiative I took. Besides this, I give blood routinely, and it's such an empowering feeling to know because of this small act of kindness I have potentially saved a life!

I usually connect everything with health and fitness, so here we go again: Studies have proven that acts of kindness, of unconditionally helping people, reduce stress and boost your immune system.

Millions and millions of people read a newspaper every day and complain about how "cruel" or "bad" the world has become. There are stories of rapes, murders, terrorist attacks, and natural calamities claiming thousands of lives. However, please note that with your complaining and criticizing, you are not doing any good for anyone. Instead my suggestion is to go out and do something about it. Be kind to a stranger, devote the time you spend reading your newspaper to your favorite charity instead.

I would like to finish this chapter and this book by quoting this prayer by Reinhold Niebuhr:

"God grant me the serenity to accept the things I cannot change, the courage to change the things I can, and the wisdom to know the difference."

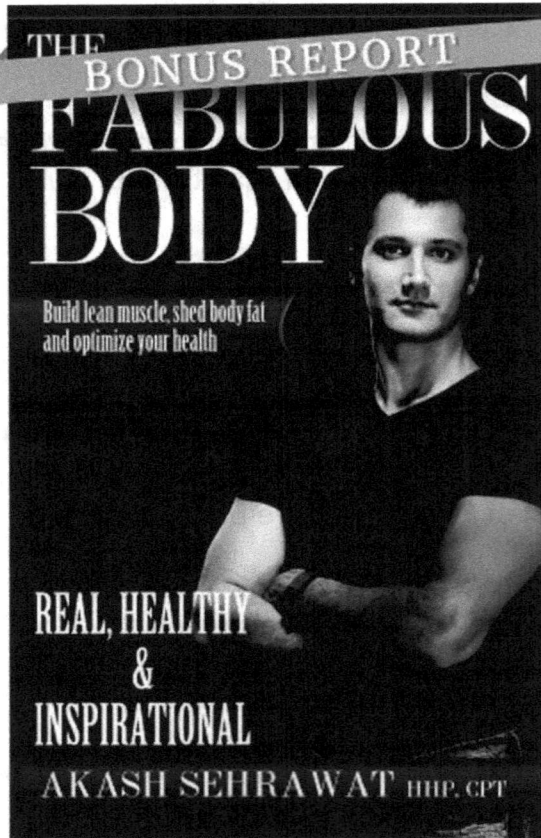

Download this FREE BONUS REPORT to get access to FBX workouts

ASK ME ANYTHING, DON'T BE SHY. ☺

Thank you for buying my book. I hope you enjoyed reading it as much as I enjoyed writing it.

Knowledge only becomes wisdom if applied. Only when you start to incorporate the information in this book, you will start to see and feel the MAGIC.

I understand that conventional wisdom can be overwhelming and confusing for most of us, and in the process of acquiring your dream physique, you will face many concerns and questions.

I care about your ultimate success, and therefore, I highly encourage you to connect with me and ask me about any doubts whatsoever. I don't charge for that, so feel free to email me:akash@fabulousbody.com

or connect with me on:

Facebook: https://www.facebook.com/fabulousbody21

Twitter: https://twitter.com/fabulousbody21

Google+: https://plus.google.com/+fabulousbody

Instagram: https://www.instagram.com/fabulousbody21/

Pinterest: https://www.pinterest.com/fabulousbody21/

Hope to hear from you.

Yours in Health,

Akash Sehrawat

Creator of fabulousbody.com

NOTE: If you enjoyed reading my book, would you do me a small favour ?

Could you write a review on Amazon about this book?

Write a review about this book on amazon.com

Write a review about this book on amazon.in

ANOTHER BOOK BY AKASH SEHRAWAT

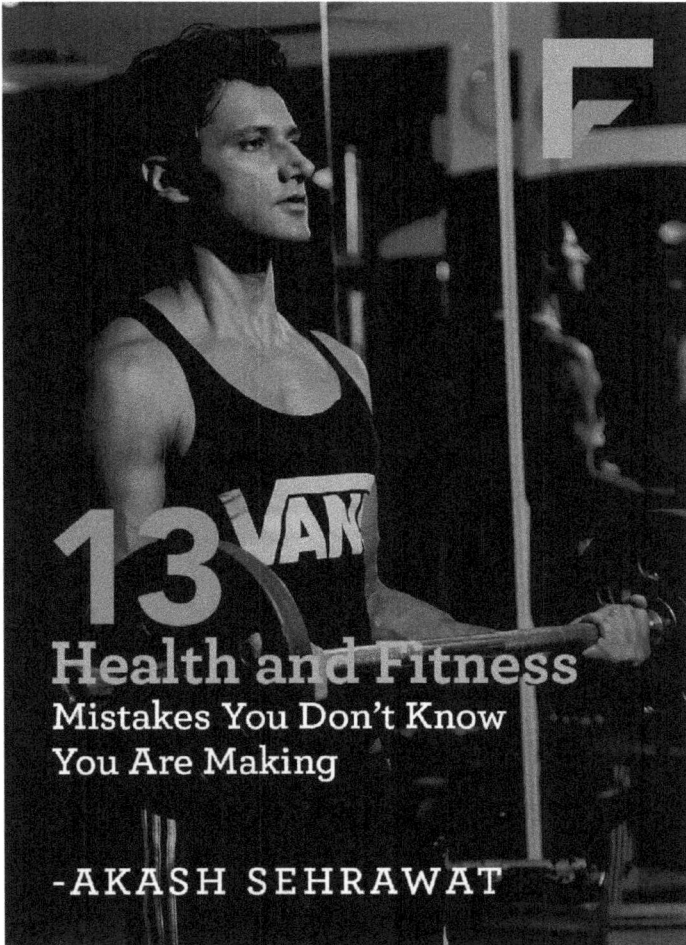

Join my weekly newsletter and get this Ebook FREE

RECOMMENDED SUPPLEMENTS

As a policy, I only recommend products that I have tried long enough to experience solid benefits.

I have been consuming Dr. Mercola products for over five years now. I usually stick with products that work, and I have never felt the need to change or try anything new. Of course, in due time, if I find something better than these products or even marginally superior (it may be in taste, quality, method of processing, sourcing of ingredients, etc.), I will surely let you know.

For now, I trust Dr. Mercola products, and my entire family uses them. (Yes, even my two-year-old boy uses Mercola baby creams!)

PRO-OPTIMAL WHEY

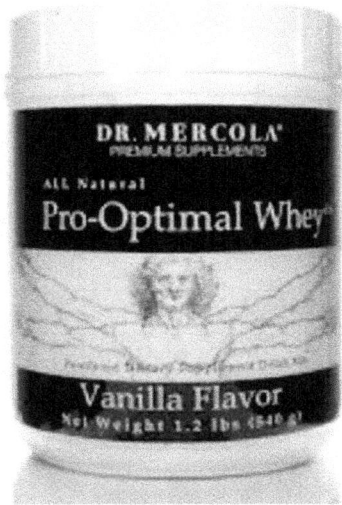

PURE POWER PROTEIN

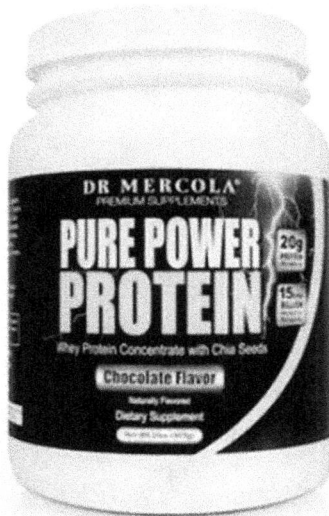

KRILL OIL

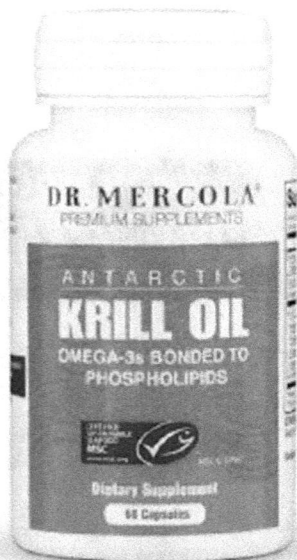

WHOLE-FOOD MULTIVITAMIN PLUS VITAL MINERALS

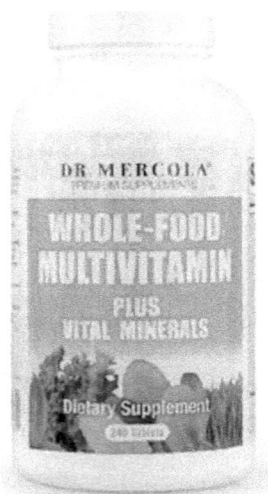

BIBLIOGRAPHY

Ideally, building a fabulous body should be a lifelong endeavor where you are constantly updating yourself with the latest research and information in the vast field of health, fitness and nutrition.

Reading this book is definitely a step forward for you, and I applaud you for taking full responsibility for your health.

I have read hundreds of books on wellness, and there are few (mentioned below) I have found to be "classics." Therefore, I highly encourage you to read them whenever you get a chance.

DR JOSEPH MERCOLA'S BOOK:

TAKE CONTROL OF YOUR HEALTH

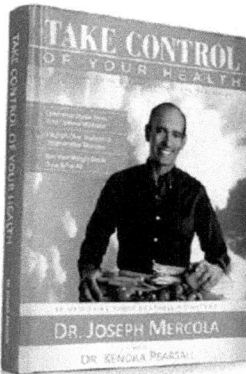

Dr. Joseph Mercola is a visionary and an intelligent and courageous doctor. He has authored three New York Times Bestsellers and has appeared on dozens of national and local news programs, including The Today Show and The Dr. Oz Show. His passion is transforming the traditional medical paradigm in the United States. He is at the forefront of the holistic health revolution and is changing the way people are thinking about health.

There are millions and millions of people who swear by his books and his website, mercola.com, where he provides tons and tons of free information to anyone who wants to take total control of his or her health.

STUART MC ROBERT'S BOOK

BRAWN

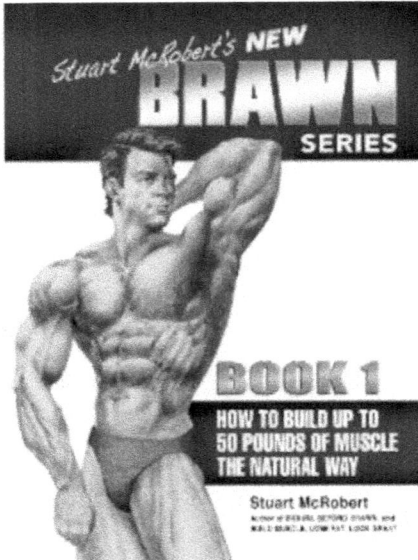

It was only after reading "Brawn" that I started appreciating the abbreviated style of training more and as a result included parallel grip deadlifts in my workout.

Stuart's books provide a wealth of information on this type of training and are must reads for anyone who wants to put on slabs of muscles in the fastest time possible and build a classic and strong physique.

REFERENCES

1) James H. O'Keefe, MD; Robert Vogel, MD; Carl J. Lavie, mD; Loren cordain, PhD, Organic Fitness: Physical activity consistent with our Hunter-Gatherer Heritage

2) Dr Zahid Naeem, MBBS, MCPS, DPH, FCPS, Professor, Vitamin D Deficiency- An Ignored Epidemic,Int J Health Sci (Qassim). 2010 Jan; 4(1): V–VI.

3) The Vitamin D Solution, by Michael F. Holick

4) Maisey DS, Vale EL, Cornelissen PL, Tovee MJ, Characteristics of male attractiveness for women, Lancet. 1999 May 1;353(9163):1500

5) Henry N. Ginsberg, Insulin resistance and cardiovascular disease, J Clin Invest. 2000 Aug 15; 106(4): 453–458

6) Scheen AJ, Pathophysiology of type 2 diabetes.

7) Jesus Millan, Xavier Pinto, Anna Munoz et al, Lipoprotein ratios: Physiological significance and clinical usefulness in cardiovascular prevention, Vasc Health Risk Manag. 2009; 5: 757–765

8) Protasio Lemos da Luz, Desiderio Favarato, et al, High Ratio of Triglycerides to HDL-Cholesterol Predicts Extensive Coronary Disease,Clinics. 2008 Aug; 63(4): 427–432

9) Mehdi H. Shishehbor, DO, Byron J. Hoogwerf, MD and Michael S. Lauer, MD,Association of Triglyceride–to–HDL Cholesterol Ratio With Heart Rate Recovery, Diabetes Care April 2004 vol. 27 no. 4 936-941

10) Seccareccia F, Menotti A,Physical activity, physical fitness and mortality in a sample of middle aged men followed-up 25 years, J Sports Med Phys Fitness. 1992 Jun;32(2):206-13

11) Hartaigh B, Jiang CQ, Bosch JA, Zhang WS, et al,, Independent and combined associations of abdominal obesity and seated resting heart rate with type 2 diabetes among older Chinese: the Guangzhou Biobank Cohort Study,Diabetes Metab Res Rev. 2011 Mar;27(3):298-306

12) https://www.ucl.ac.uk/news/news-articles/0908/09080401

13) E. G. Trapp, D. J. Chisholm, J. Freund, and S. H. Boutcher, "The effects of high-intensity intermittent exercise training on fat loss and fasting insulin levels of young women," International Journal of Obesity, vol. 32, no. 4, pp. 684–691, 2008

14) Schuenke MD, Mikat RP, Mc Bride JM, Effect of an acute period of resistance exercise on excess post-exercise oxygen consumption: implications for body mass management, Eur J Appl Physiol. 2002 Mar;86(5):411-7. Epub 2002 Jan 29

15) Bales CW, Kraus WE, Caloric restriction: implications for human cardiometabolic health,J Cardiopulm Rehabil Prev. 2013 Jul-Aug;33(4):201-8

16) Mattson MP, Wan R, Beneficial effects of intermittent fasting and caloric restriction on the cardiovascular and cerebrovascular systems, J Nutr Biochem. 2005 Mar;16(3):129-37

17) Varady KA, Hellerstein MK, Alternate-day fasting and chronic disease prevention: a review of human and animal trials, Am J Clin Nutr. 2007 Jul;86(1):7-13

18) Johnstone A, Fasting for weight loss: an effective strategy or latest dieting trend? Int J Obes (Lond). 2015 May;39(5):727-33

19) Cameron JD, Cyr MJ, Doucet E, Increased meal frequency does not promote greater weight loss in subjects who were prescribed an 8-week

equi-energetic energy-restricted diet, Br J Nutr. 2010 Apr;103(8):1098-101

20) Rooney, KJ, Herbert, RD, and Balnave, RJF. Fatigue contributes to the strength training stimulus. Med Sci Sport Exerc 26: 1160–1164, 1994.

21) Schott, J, McCully, K, and Rutherford, OM. The role of metabolites in strength training. II. Short versus long isometric contractions. Eur J Appl Physiol 71: 337–341, 1995.

22) Smith,RC and Rutherford,OM. The role of metabolites in strength training. A comparison of eccentric and concentric contractions. Eur J Appl Physiol Occup Physiol 71: 332–336, 1995.

23) Folland, JP, Irish, CS, Roberts, JC, Tarr, JE, and Jones, DA. Fatigue is not a necessary stimulus for strength gains during resistance training. Br J Sports Med 36: 370–373, 2002.

24) Suga,T,Okita,K,Morita,N,Yokota,T,Hirabayashi,K,Horiuchi,M, Takada, S, Takahashi, T, Omokawa, M, Kinugawa, S, and Tsutsui, H. Intramuscular metabolism during low-intensity resistance exercise with blood flow restriction. J Appl Physiol 106: 1119–1124, 2009.

25) Tesch, PA, Colliander, EB, and Kaiser, P. Muscle metabolism during intense, heavy-resistance exercise. Eur J Appl Physiol Occup Physiol 55: 362–366, 1986.

26) Kraemer, WJ and Ratamess, NA. Hormonal responses and adaptations to resistance exercise and training. Sport Med 35: 339–361, 2005.

27) Y. Takahashi, D.M. Kipnis, and W.H. Daughaday, Growth hormone secretion during sleep, J Clin Invest. 1968 Sep; 47(9): 2079–2090

28) Welle S, Thornton C, Statt M, McHenry B, Growth hormone increases muscle mass and strength but does not rejuvenate myofibrillar

protein synthesis in healthy subjects over 60 years old, J Clin Endocrinol Metab. 1996 Sep;81(9):3239-43

29) C P Velloso, Regulation of muscle mass by growth hormone and IGF-1, Br J Pharmacol. 2008 Jun; 154(3): 557–568

30) Tarnopolsky MA, Atkinson SA, McDougall JD, et al, Evaluation of protein requirements for trained strength athletes, J Appl Physiol (1985). 1992 Nov;73(5):1986-95

31) Kreider RB, Campbell B, Protein for exercise and recovery, Phys Sportsmed. 2009 Jun;37(2):13-21

32) Lemon PW, Beyond the zone: protein needs of active individuals, J Am Coll Nutr. 2000 Oct;19(5 Suppl):513S-521S

33) Lemon PW, Tarnopolsky MA, McDougall JD, et al, Protein requirements and muscle mass/strength changes during intensive training in novice bodybuilders, J Appl Physiol (1985). 1992 Aug;73(2):767-75

34) James H. o'Keefe, mD; Robert Vogel, mD; carl J. Lavie, mD; Loren cordain, PhD, Organic Fitness: Physical activity consistent with our Hunter-Gatherer Heritage

35) http://www.acsm.org/about-acsm/media-room/news-releases/2011/08/01/acsm-issues-new-recommendations-on-quantity-and-quality-of-exercise

36) Judge LW, Burke JR, The effect of recovery time on strength performance following a high-intensity bench press workout in males and females,Int J Sports Physiol Perform. 2010 Jun;5(2):184-96

37) Orzel-Gryglewska J, Consequences of sleep deprivation,Int J Occup Med Environ Health. 2010;23(1):95-114

38) Robillard R, Prince F, Boissonneault M, Filipini D, Carrier J, Effects of increased homeostatic sleep pressure on postural control and their

modulation by attentional resources, Clin Neurophysiol. 2011 Sep;122(9):1771-8

39) Colten HR, Altevogt BM, Sleep Disorders and Sleep Deprivation: An Unmet Public Health Problem, Washington (DC): National Academies Press (US); 2006. 2, Sleep Physiology

40) Morton SK, Whitehead JR, Brinkert RH, Caine DJ, Resistance training vs. static stretching: effects on flexibility and strength, J Strength Cond Res. 2011 Dec;25(12):3391-8

41) http://www.exrx.net/Calculators/OneRepMax.html

42) Rhea MR, Alvar BA, Burkett LN, Ball SD, A meta-analysis to determine the dose responses for strength development, Med Sci Sports Exerc. 2003 Mar;35(3):456-64

43) https://www.acsm.org/docs/brochures/high-intensity-interval-training.pdf

44) Valerie F Gladwell, Daniel K Brown, Carly Wood, et al, The great outdoors: how a green exercise environment can benefit all, Extrem Physiol Med. 2013; 2: 3

45) Stephan H. Boutcher, High-Intensity Intermittent Exercise and Fat Loss,J Obes. 2011; 2011: 868305

46) Jansson E, Esbjornsson M, Holm I, Jacobs I, Increase in the proportion of fast-twitch muscle fibres by sprint training in males, Acta Physiol Scand. 1990 Nov;140(3):359-63

47) Kristian Karstoft MD, Kamilla Winding, MSC, et al, The Effects of Free-Living Interval-Walking Training on Glycemic Control, Body Composition, and Physical Fitness in Type 2 Diabetic Patients, Diabetes Care February 2013 vol. 36 no. 2 228-236

48) http://acsm.ideafit.com/acsm/acsm-september-october-2014-health-fitness-journal

49) Wilmot EG, Edwardson CL, Achana FA, Davies MJ, et al, Sedentary time in adults and the association with diabetes, cardiovascular disease and death: systematic review and meta-analysis, Diabetologia. 2012 Nov;55(11):2895-905

50) Rory Heath, Sitting Ducks—Sedentary Behaviour and its risks: Part One of a Two Part Series, 21st Jan, 15 by BJSM

51) http://www.thewalkingsite.com

52) Watkins J. Structure and function of the musculoskeletal system. Champaign, IL: Human Kinetics; 1999

53) http://www.nytimes.com/1999/05/25/health/95-regain-lost-weight-or-do-they.html?pagewanted=all&_r=0

54) Blumenthal, Daniel M, Gold, Mark S, Neurobiology of food addiction, July 2010 - Volume 13 - Issue 4 - p 359—365

55) http://rawfoodsos.com/2011/12/22/the-truth-about-ancel-keys-weve-all-got-it-wrong/

56) Patty W Siri-Tarino, Qi Sun, Frank B Hu, et al, Meta-analysis of prospective cohort studies evaluating the association of saturated fat with cardiovascular disease,Am J Clin Nutr. 2010 Mar; 91(3): 535–546

57) Aseem Malhotra interventional cardiology specialist registrar, Croydon University Hospital, London, Saturated Fat is not the major issue, BMJ 2013;347:f6340

58) Rajiv Chowdhary, MD, PhD, Samantha Warnakula, MPhil, Setor Kunutsor, MD, et al,Association of Dietary, Circulating, and Supplement Fatty Acids With Coronary Risk: A Systematic Review and Meta-analysis, Ann Intern Med. 2014;160(6):398-406

59) Janice K. Kiecolt-Glaser, Martha A Belury, Rebecca Andridge, et al, Omega-3 Supplementation Lowers Inflammation in Healthy Middle-Aged and Older Adults: A Randomized Controlled Trial, Brain Behav Immun. 2012 Aug; 26(6): 988—995

60) Nestel P, Clifton P, C, et al, Indications for Omega-3 Long Chain Polyunsaturated Fatty Acid in the Prevention and Treatment of Cardiovascular Disease, Heart Lung Circ. 2015 Aug;24(8):769-79

61) Bauer I, Hughes M, Rowsell R, et al, Omega-3 supplementation improves cognition and modifies brain activation in young adults, Hum Psychopharmacol. 2014 Mar;29(2):133-44

62) Stonehouse W, Conlon CA, et al, DHA supplementation improved both memory and reaction time in healthy young adults: a randomized controlled trial, Am J Clin Nutr. 2013 May;97(5):1134-43

63) Vinot N, Jouin M, et al,Omega-3 fatty acids from fish oil lower anxiety, improve cognitive functions and reduce spontaneous locomotor activity in a non-human primate, PLoS One. 2011;6(6):e20491

64) McNamara RK, Long-chain omega-3 fatty acid deficiency in mood disorders: rationale for treatment and prevention,Curr Drug Discov Technol. 2013 Sep;10(3):233-44.

65) Micheal H Bloch, Jonas Hannestad, Omega-3 Fatty Acids for the Treatment of Depression: Systematic Review and Meta-Analysis, Mol Psychiatry. 2012 Dec; 17(12): 1272—1282

66) Giuseppe Grosso, Fabio Galvano, Stefano Marventano, et al, Omega-3 Fatty Acids and Depression: Scientific Evidence and Biological Mechanisms, Oxid Med Cell Longev. 2014; 2014: 313570

67) Qi Sun, Jing Ma, Hannia Campos, et al, A Prospective Study of Trans Fatty Acids in Erythrocytes and Risk of Coronary Heart Disease, Circulation. 2007; 115: 1858-1865

68) Tarnopolsky MA, Atkinson SA, McDougall JD, et al, Evaluation of protein requirements for trained strength athletes, J Appl Physiol (1985). 1992 Nov;73(5):1986-95

69) Kreider RB, Campbell B, Protein for exercise and recovery, Phys Sportsmed. 2009 Jun;37(2):13-21

70) Lemon PW, Beyond the zone: poten needs of active individuals, J Am Coll Nutr. 2000 Oct;19(5 Suppl):513S-521S

71) Lemon PW, Tarnopolsky MA, McDougall JD, et al, Protein requirements and muscle mass/strength changes during intensive training in novice bodybuilders, J Appl Physiol (1985). 1992 Aug;73(2):767-75

72) Martin WF, Armstrong LE, Rodriguez NR, Dietary protein intake and renal function, Nutr Metab (Lond). 2005 Sep 20;2:25

73) Pecoits-Filho R, Dietary protein intake and kidney disease in Western Diet, Contrib Nephrol. 2007;155:102-12

74) Blum M, Averbuch M, Wolman Y, Aviram A, Protein intake and kidney function in humans: its effect on 'normal aging', Arch Intern Med. 1989 Jan;149(1):211-2

75) Frank B. Hu, Vasanti S. Malik, Sugar-sweetened beverages and risk of obesity and type 2 diabetes: Epidemiologic evidence, Physiol Behav. 2010 Apr 26; 100(1): 47–54.

76) Lenny R. Vartanian, Marlene B. Schwartz, et al, Effects of Soft Drink Consumption on Nutrition and Health: A Systematic Review and Meta-Analysis, Am J Public Health. 2007 April; 97(4): 667–675

77) Apovian CM, Sugar-sweetened soft drinks, obesity, and type 2 diabetes, JAMA. 2004 Aug 25;292(8):978-9

78) Scott M Grundy, Hypertriglyceridemia, insulin resistance, and the metabolic syndrome, the american journal of cardiology, May 13, 1999, Volume 83, Issue 9, Supplement 2, Page 25—29

79) Matthias B. Schulze, Joann E. Manson, David s. Ludwig, et al, Sugar-Sweetened Beverages, Weight Gain, and Incidence of Type 2 Diabetes in Young and Middle-Aged Women, JAMA. 2004;292(8):927-934

80) M L Slattery, J Benson, T D Berry, et al, Dietary sugar and colon cancer, Cancer Epidemiol Biomarkers Prev September 1997 6; 677

81) Roberd M. Bostick, John D. Potter, Lawrence H. Kushi, Sugar, meat, and fat intake, and non-dietary risk factors for colon cancer incidence in Iowa women (United States), Cancer Causes & Control January 1994, Volume 5, Issue 1, pp 38-52

82) Stephen Seely, David F Horrobin, Diet and breast cancer: The possible connection with sugar consumption, Volume 11, Issue 3, July 1983, Pages 319-327

83) Nils Halberg, Morten Henriksen, Nathalie Soderhamn, et al, Effect of intermittent fasting and refeeding on insulin action in healthy men Journal of Applied Physiology Published 1 December 2005 Vol. 99 no. 6, 2128-2136

84) Bales CW, Kraus WE, Caloric restriction: implications for human cardiometabolic health,J Cardiopulm Rehabil Prev. 2013 Jul-Aug;33(4):201-8

85) Mattson MP, Wan R, Beneficial effects of intermittent fasting and caloric restriction on the cardiovascular and cerebrovascular systems,J Nutr Biochem. 2005 Mar;16(3):129-37

86) Varady KA, Hellerstein MK, Alternate-day fasting and chronic disease prevention: a review of human and animal trials.Am J Clin Nutr. 2007 Jul;86(1):7-13

87) Horne BD, May HT, Anderson JL, et al, Usefulness of routine periodic fasting to lower risk of coronary artery disease in patients undergoing coronary angiography,

88) http://www.sciencedaily.com/releases/2011/04/110403090259.htm

89) http://www.consumerreports.org/cro/2012/04/protein-drinks/index.htm

90) http://www.naturalnews.com/041510_Acesulfame-K_methylene_chloride_carcinogen.html

91) http://articles.mercola.com/sites/articles/archive/2009/02/10/new-study-of-splenda-reveals-shocking-information-about-potential-harmful-effects.aspx

92) http://www.prevention.com/food/healthy-eating-tips/health-risks-sucralose

93) E. Patterson, R. Wall, G. F. Fitzgerald, et al, Health Implications of High Dietary Omega-6 Polyunsaturated Fatty Acids, J Nutr Metab. 2012; 2012: 539426

94) http://www.bmj.com/press-releases/2013/02/04/study-raises-questions-about-dietary-fats-and-heart-disease-guidance

95) R J. Moon, N. C. Harvey, S. M. Robinson, et al, Maternal Plasma Polyunsaturated Fatty Acid Status in Late Pregnancy Is Associated with Offspring Body Composition in Childhood, The Journal of Clinical Endocrinology & Metabolism, Volume 98, Issue 1

96) Simopoulos AP, The importance of the ratio of omega-6/omega-3 essential fatty acids, Biomed Pharmacother. 2002 Oct;56(8):365-79

97) Janice K. Kiecolt-Glaser, Martha A. Belury, et al, Omega-3 Supplementation Lowers Inflammation in Healthy Middle-Aged and Older Adults: A Randomized Controlled Trial, Brain Behav Immun. 2012 Aug; 26(6): 988–995.

98) http://umm.edu/health/medical/altmed/supplement/omega3-fatty-acids

99) http://articles.mercola.com/sites/articles/archive/2014/02/10/krill-oil-supplementation.aspx

100) http://www.mreassociates.org/pages/ama_speaks_out.html

101) J. Micheal Gaziano, Howard D. Sesso, et al, Multivitamins in the Prevention of Cancer in Men, The Physicians' Health Study II Randomized Controlled Trial, November 14, 2012, Vol 308, No. 18

102) Regan L Bailey, Tala H Faakhouri, et al, Multivitamin-Mineral Use Is Associated with Reduced Risk of Cardiovascular Disease Mortality among Women in the United States, First published January 7, 2015

103) Garland CF, Gorham ED, et al, Vitamin D for cancer prevention: global perspective, Ann Epidemiol. 2009 Jul;19(7):468-83

104) http://orthomolecular.org/resources/omns/v11n01.shtml

www.ingramcontent.com/pod-product-compliance
Lightning Source LLC
Chambersburg PA
CBHW060453280326
41933CB00014B/2741